Conversations with My Kids
30 Essential Family Discussions for the Digital Age

Rising Parent Media, LLC

23 22 21 20 19 1 2 3 4 5

ISBN: 978-1-7336046-9-7 (paperback)

The paper used in this publication meets the minimum requirements of the American National Standard for Information Sciences—Permanence of Paper for Printed Library Materials, ANSI Z39.48-1992.

FOR GREAT RESOURCES AND INFORMATION,
FOLLOW US ON OUR SOCIAL MEDIA OUTLETS:

Facebook: www.facebook.com/educateempowerkids/
Twitter: @EduEmpowerKids
Pinterest: pinterest.com/educateempower/
Instagram: Eduempowerkids

Thank you to the following people for their support during this project:

Amanda Kimball, Mary Bassett
Robert Jensen, Ph.D
Kyle Roberts, MA, Cliff Park, MBA, Byran Korth, Ph.D, and Tim Rarick, Ph.D

CONVERSATIONS WITH MY KIDS

30 ESSENTIAL FAMILY DISCUSSIONS FOR PARENTING IN THE DIGITAL AGE

EDUCATE AND EMPOWER KIDS WOULD LIKE TO ACKNOWLEDGE THE FOLLOWING PEOPLE WHO CONTRIBUTED TIME, TALENTS, AND ENERGY TO THIS PUBLICATION:

Dina Alexander, MS
Melody Bergman
Jenny Webb, MA

DESIGN AND ILLUSTRATION BY:

Jera Mehrdad
Jenny Webb, MA

OUR GOAL:

TO PROVIDE TOOLS THAT FACILITATE AMAZING CONVERSATIONS TO HELP YOU FORM A DEEPER CONNECTION WITH YOUR KIDS AND STRENGTHEN YOUR ENTIRE FAMILY

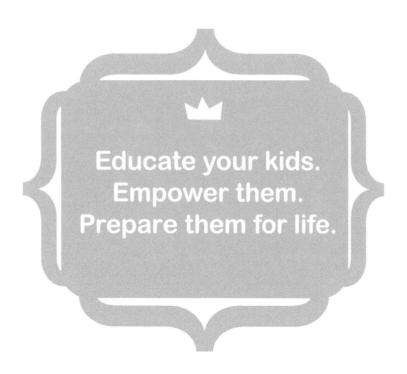

**Educate your kids.
Empower them.
Prepare them for life.**

INTRODUCTION

The world is changing around us at an ever increasing speed. New technology and massive amounts of readily available information can sometimes inspire us, but are often empty or meaningless. This is why it's imperative for us as parents (and caring adults) to be empathetic listeners and a source of useful, worthwhile information for our children. We must teach our kids how to find answers to their questions and how to know the difference between right and wrong, between truth and deception.

Every kid is faced with a huge variety of pressures on every side: to conform, to lose hope, to give up, to push down feelings, to escape hard work and challenges, or to avoid following one's heart and mind, among others.

We can help our kids face these challenges by connecting with them in meaningful conversations about important topics, including the struggles they face or will face in the future. We have provided thirty essential conversations for your family to engage with. Please feel free to adapt these simple discussions to fit your needs and the needs of your children.

USING THIS BOOK

Connecting with our kids begins with simple, daily interactions. Use these simple conversation starters to talk about deep issues. Have fun as you tackle these topics, even the heavy ones. Find the humor in tough talks and learn to lighten up as you help your kids face life's challenges.

You do not need to be an expert in any of the topics we have provided in order to have stimulating, relevant conversations. This book is simply a tool to spark great discussions, encourage closeness, and strengthen your family. Remember, the questions provided do not necessarily have right or wrong answers. If you don't know the answer to a question, explore the topic with your child—seek out their opinion and experience.

Don't worry if you don't have time for a lengthy family discussion for every topic in this book. Even if you only have five minutes, that will work! Hit the highlights, ask a couple of questions, and know that you can return to the topic later. The point is to let your kids know you care about them enough to connect.

Lastly, as the greek philosopher Epictetus noted, "We were given two ears and one mouth so we could listen twice as much as we speak." Adults: practice this principle when having these talks with your kids.

NEW WORDS: *We will be introducing several topics that may be new to your kids throughout the book. To facilitate discussion, we have* **bolded** *many of these terms. Definitions of these words can be found at the end of the book, in the Glossary.*

FOR ADDITIONAL IDEAS AND INFORMATION, COME VISIT US AT WWW.EDUCATEEMPOWERKIDS.ORG

TABLE OF CONTENTS

TECHNOLOGY

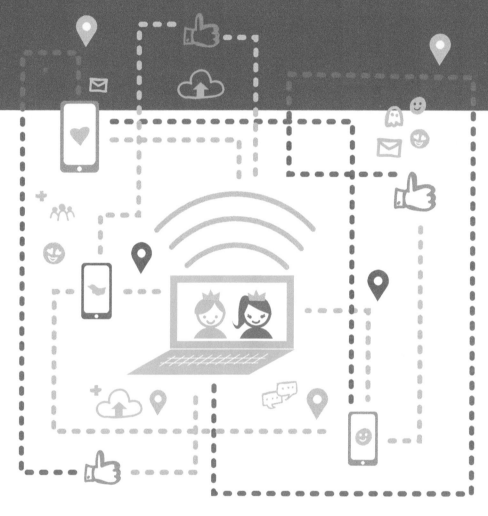

We have created a world full of technology and every human is affected by its power and influence—especially kids! Each time we text, send an email, post on social media, interact with others in a game, or create a new piece of technology, we create ripples.

All of our actions online and in "real life" create ripples (small waves of change) around us.

The topics in this section provide a great opportunity to talk about the enormous power and responsibility each of us hold within our smartphones and other tech we use. Use the following questions and activities to discuss the great potential available in technology and how we can practice healthy tech boundaries.

1. USING TECHNOLOGY FOR GOOD

We can create amazing ripples (small waves of change) when we use technology for good. This idea is often referred to as **positive digital citizenship**—using tech to enhance your family, school, and community through **tolerance**, kindness, authenticity, and ingenuity.

Examples of using tech for good include: posting an uplifting quote, complimenting someone on social media or in a text, cheering someone up with a joke or funny meme, creating a petition on a website like change.org to help make a difference in your community, sharing useful, true information online, standing up for someone who is being treated poorly, using an app or online forum to organize local people to volunteer to serve others, or starting an online movement to bring awareness to an important issue.

However you choose to use technology, make sure you are the same person online, offline, and everywhere in between, whether you think someone is watching or not.

- -

DISCUSSION QUESTIONS

👑 What are some things you can do with a smartphone, tablet, or computer?

👑 What can you learn, teach others, and create?

👑 What are some ways we can help and uplift others and create positive ripples with technology?

👑 Are you the same person online that you are in "real life"?

👑 Technology has made it easier to reach out to presidents, senators, mayors, favorite authors, experts, celebrities, and other influential people through email or social media. Who would you like to connect with and why?

👑 Websites, forums, and social media make it possible to connect with organizations and people who care about the same things you might care about (animals, sports, the environment, assisting refugees, etc.).

👑 What groups and individuals would you like to join or learn more about?

👑 Technology is powerful! How can you change the world using technology?

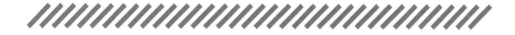

ACTIVITIES

Post Something Positive
Set a goal to use your smartphone to lift and build up others. Create a plan that will help you to remember to text or post positive, uplifting comments to friends and family members on a daily basis.

Petition for Change
Create a petition on change.org to create a crosswalk for a busy street, add a playground to a park, eliminate plastic bags in your local community, or any other project you feel will create positive change in your local community.

Commit to Stand Up
Learn how to stop online bullying on becauseofyou.org. Make a commitment to be a good digital citizen, and stand up for the victim if you see someone being mistreated online.

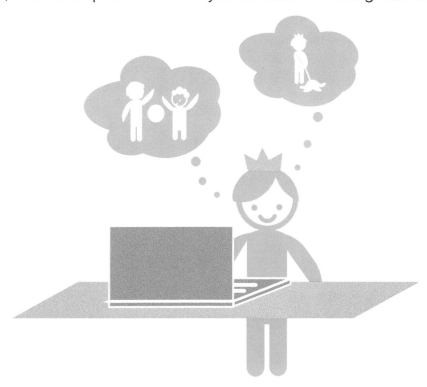

CITATIONS/RESOURCES

Alexander, D. (2017). *Noah's New Phone: A Story About Using Technology for Good.* (J. Webb, M. Warner, and T. Mattsson, eds.). Rising Parent Media.

Educate and Empower Kids. (n.d.). Lesson: Using Technology for Good. Retrieved from https://educateempowerkids.org/wp-content/uploads/2016/09/TechnologyForGood_LessonPlan.pdf.

Farrin, F. and M. Bergman. (n.d.). 10 Ways Kids Can Use Technology for Good. Retrieved from https://educateempowerkids.org/4381-2/.

Hawks, H. (n.d.). 5 Ways Kids Can Use Smartphones for Good. Retrieved from https://educateempowerkids.org/5-ways-kids-can-use-smartphones-good/.

2. SCREENS EVERYWHERE

Media messages are very powerful and we are surrounded by them. On every screen we look at, we are engaging with a type of media whether it is a movie, an app, a book, a website, a video game, or an online advertisement.

Because we spend so much time with phones, laptops, and other devices, it is vital that we understand the messages we are consuming and set firm, realistic boundaries about how much time we spend with screens.

Even when we are doing useful, necessary tasks with screens like homework, research, reading the news, emailing, etc., we should be aware of how the hours of screen time are affecting us.

- -

DISCUSSION QUESTIONS

- When we are in front of a screen, especially our phones, are we being **deliberate** and **intentional** with our actions or are we bored, finding it easy to fill up time by simply scrolling through a feed?

- Are you able to complete a job or finish a homework assignment without checking your phone several times?

- What is a healthy amount of time to spend in front of a screen each day?

- What is an appropriate age for kids to receive a smartphone?

- If you have a phone, what are some things you use it for?

- What are some ways your siblings and parents use their phones?

- How much texting or posting on social media in one day is too much?

- Do you have "device free" time? For example, do you put phones and tablets away at dinner time?

Much of our screen time is media-based—this includes social media like Facebook or Instagram.

- How does media affect our choices or shape our beliefs, political views, and attitudes?

- Can you recognize the signs in yourself that most people exhibit when spending too much time on screens (irritability, withdrawal, lack of attention, problems with impulse control)?

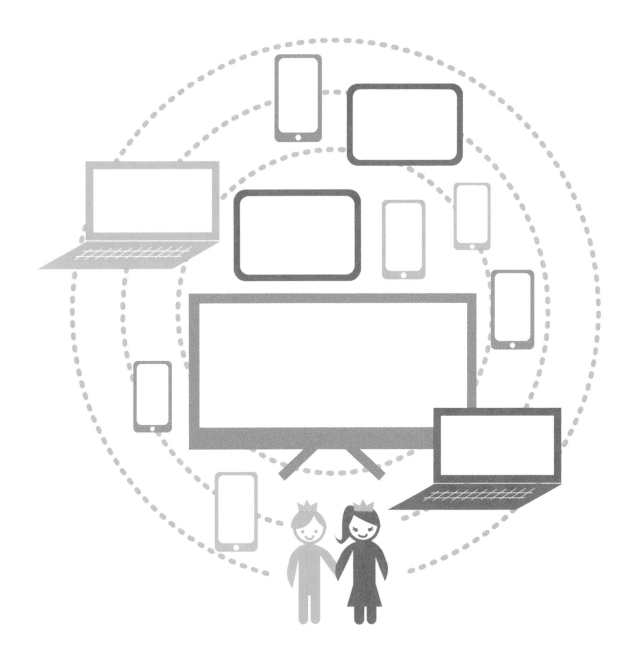

STAYING SAFE

With technology being easily accessible to kids through smartphones, tablets, and computers, they are also easily exposed to violence, sexual imagery, and online predators.

> ♛ Is your family having open conversations about online safety and some of the dangers encountered on the internet?

Predators will always "go" where kids are, and today, kids are online.

> ♛ How can we protect ourselves, our kids, and our personal information from predators? How else do we stay safe online?

GAMING

Kids and adults spend a lot of time playing video games on smartphones, tablets, and computers.

- Can lessons be learned while gaming?

- Is there value in construction-based games like Minecraft?

- Can gaming together with siblings or family members build family relationships?

- Is gaming a positive coping skill (a way to relax or process stress)?

- -

ACTIVITY

Break It Down
Media's messages can be **deconstructed**. This means we can break apart their elements to determine the real message. This can be done with ads, TV shows, YouTube videos, or basically anything you can find on a screen!

Look at an advertisement (an online ad, or an ad from a magazine) together and ask the following questions:

- What methods were used in this ad to get our attention? Why was this ad made?

- What is the overall message? What is the underlying or hidden message?

- How does this advertisement make you feel?

- -

CITATIONS/RESOURCES

Alexander, D. (2017). *Noah's New Phone: A Story About Using Technology for Good*. (J. Webb, M. Warner, and T. Mattsson, eds.). Rising Parent Media.

Alexander, D. (2018). Petra's Power to See: A Media Literacy Adventure. (M. Bergman, ed.). Rising Parent Media.

Andrews, C. (n.d.). Creating a Media Guideline for Your Family. Retrieved from https://educateempowerkids.org/creating-media-guideline-family-2/.

Educate and Empower Kids. (n.d.). Lesson: Using Technology for Good. Retrieved from https://educateempowerkids.org/wp-content/uploads/2016/09/TechnologyForGood_LessonPlan.pdf.

Robinson, A. (n.d.). The Danger with Using Screens as a Digital Pacifier. Retrieved from https://educateempowerkids.org/danger-using-screens-digital-pacifier/.

Spears, M. (n.d.). Tech Over-Use and Lazy Parenting: A Deadly Combination. Retrieved from https://educateempowerkids.org/tech-use-lazy-parenting-deadly-combination/.

3. SOCIAL MEDIA

Social media is a powerful tool! It forms a unique opportunity where we can actually *create* media and share a message. We can use this power to reach hundreds or thousands of people. We can choose to tear people down or lift them up.

Social media includes websites and apps that people over the age of 13 use to share information and develop personal and professional relationships. Facebook, Google+, Instagram, Pinterest, Snapchat, and Twitter are examples of social media.

Our actions online and in "real life" create ripples (small waves of change) around us. Make sure you are creating positive ripples by complimenting others on social media, being respectful even when you disagree with someone, standing up for others, reporting **bullying**, and listening to others' opinions.

DISCUSSION QUESTIONS

- What is an appropriate age for kids to start using social media?
- What are some examples of appropriate behavior on social media?
- What behavior is not okay?

WHEN POSTING, ASK YOURSELF:

- When I post on social media, am I being clear in my message?
- Do I really understand the issue or concern I am posting about? Am I being true to myself?
- Am I being authentic? Is my message helpful?
- Is my message kind? How will my message be received?
- Is this something I want on the internet FOREVER?

Positive Posts Challenge
Challenge your family to make their social media interactions more positive. Set a goal to post only positive things for one week. Encourage family members to share uplifting, informative, or humorous examples.

Share Awareness
Share a video or post that draws awareness to the plight of people struggling (refugees, the homeless, hungry children, etc.).

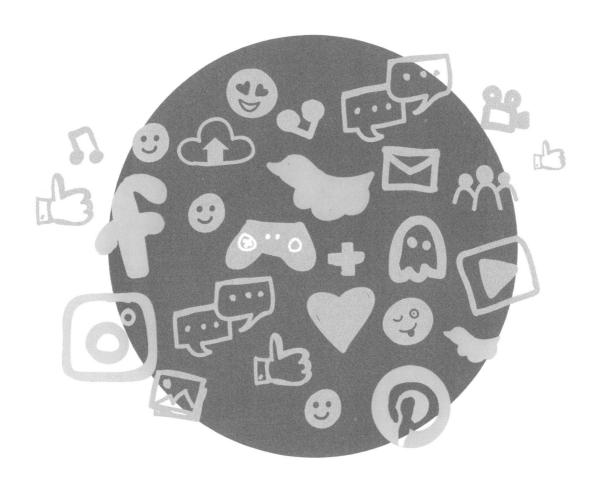

CITATIONS/RESOURCES

Alexander, D. (2018). *Petra's Power to See: A Media Literacy Adventure*. (M. Bergman, ed.). Rising Parent Media.

Educate and Empower Kids. (2018). Social Media and Teens: The Ultimate Guide to Keeping Kids Safe Online. Retrieved from https://educateempowerkids.org/5280-2/.

Alexander, D. (n.d.). What Parents Need to Know About Their Kids and Social Media. [Video File]. Retrieved from

https://www.mormonchannel.org/watch/series/gospel-solutions-for-families/what-parents-need-to-know-about-their-kids-and-social-media.

4. ALGORITHMS AND ARTIFICIAL INTELLIGENCE (AI)

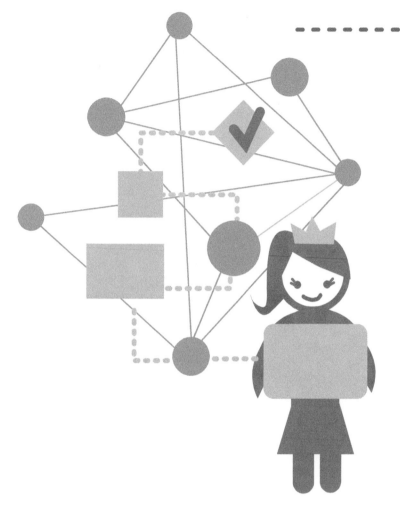

Algorithms provide a series of instructions that the computer follows to arrive at an answer, and they underlie all of our technology. When you type a search into Google, it uses a very sophisticated algorithm that determines which pages on the internet are relevant to your search and ranks them based on how relevant and reputable they are.

The algorithm that recommends connections on social media (like the "People You May Know" recommendations on Facebook or suggested people to follow on Instagram) works by calculating your degrees of separation from other users. If you are friends with Amy and Amy is friends with Ben, Facebook assumes that you might know Ben as well and recommends him as a potential connection.

When you use Amazon or Netflix, they recommend purchases or other shows you might be interested in based on a collaborative filtering algorithm that tries to predict what users will like based on the choices of other users with similar taste profiles.

Algorithms used by Facebook, Amazon, Google, and other websites give us the illusion of choice. We may think we are choosing products or websites from a random collection, but we are not! Actually, the items and people and search results we see online are there for a specific purpose. A computer program has determined what we are most likely to click on so that we will make a purchase or stay on a website.

Algorithms are a type of **artificial intelligence**. Self-driving cars, Amazon's Alexa, internet radio like Spotify and Pandora, online games, and YouTube are all examples of artificial intelligence (usually using algorithms to function).

👑 What are the benefits and the problems with the "illusion of choice" we encounter in social media, Google, Amazon, and other websites?

👑 Does it matter that we are not making a totally free or open choice when we're choosing games on a gaming site or shopping for a certain product on Amazon or other shopping websites? (Do you ever worry that "Siri" and "Alexa" are listening to everything we say?)

👑 What would our online lives look like if we really had random options on Facebook, Amazon, and Google?

👑 Should we be concerned that powerful companies like Amazon, Facebook, and Google have so much control over the choices we are presented with online?

👑 What do you think your future will be like if algorithms are even more involved in your life (i.e. medical diagnoses, dating apps, social media "friends," job hunting online, etc.)?

DISCUSSION FOR OLDER KIDS & TEENS

In the old days many people were concerned that the government would be able to control its citizens by closely monitoring and spying on their activities. Now many people are concerned that large corporations, including those that sell to and host sites for children, are monitoring every action people make online and *selling* that data.

What might be some of the potential problems with corporations monitoring all of our online behavior, including our interactions with ANY device that can connect to the internet, such as refrigerators, televisions, phones, and even robotic vacuums?

Can individuals, a community, or a nation truly have free speech if communication happens through a third-party company whose focus is making money (like Facebook or Google)?

CITATIONS/RESOURCES

Galloway, S. (Oct. 2017). How Amazon, Apple, Facebook, and Google Manipulate Our Emotions [Video File]. Retrieved from https://www.ted.com/talks/scott_galloway_how_amazon_apple_facebook_and_google_manipulate_our_emotions#t-42838.

Greene, T. (Aug. 2, 2018). A Beginner's Guide to AI: Algorithms. Retrieved from https://thenextweb.com/artificial intelligence/2018/08/02/a-beginners-guide-to-ai-algorithms/.

Tufekci, Z. (Sep. 2017). We're Building a Dystopia Just to Make People Click on Ads [Video File]. Retrieved from https://www.ted.com/talks/zeynep_tufekci_we_re_building_a_dystopia_just_to_make_people_click_on_ads.

Tynker: Coding for Kids. (Mar. 26, 2016). Understanding the Basic Algorithms that Power Your Digital Life. Retrieved from https://www.tynker.com/blog/articles/ideas-and-tips/understanding-the-basic-algorithms-that-power-your-digital-life/.

5. CHANGING TECHNOLOGIES

Sometimes it feels like technology is moving and changing very quickly. It used to be that when something was invented, it remained important and unique for many years (like radio and television). Now new technology can become outdated or lose popularity with a few years, months, or even weeks.

Some people feel threatened by new technology. They may also feel overwhelmed trying to keep up with the changes in how we communicate, build relationships, and complete work-related tasks using technology. However, there are many benefits to using smartphones, wireless internet, streaming video services, video chat, online shopping, apps for everything, virtual reality, and more. Technology makes it easier to communicate with family and friends, connect with people all over the world, build business relationships, map a trip, be entertained, and get information instantly.

But we should also take the time to evaluate our tech use and determine whether or not certain technologies are useful in our lives and in our homes. We need to be vigilant concerning every technology that we interact with, how much information the technology collects, and who it shares that information with.

We need to be **deliberate** in our daily tech use, especially when participating on social media. Most importantly, we should take inventory regarding how much time we spend with screens and how much time we spend with people in face-to-face experiences. Stop and make sure all the awesome technology the world has to offer is not robbing you of your humanity.

- -

DISCUSSION QUESTIONS

- Everyone seems to own a smartphone. What are the potential benefits with so many people owning smartphones? (Ease in communication, use of GPS to map a trip, get information quickly, etc.)

- What are the potential setbacks with so many people owning smartphones? (Fewer in-person conversations, loss of **empathy**, inability to wait, loss of patience, etc.)

- Why are some people afraid of new technologies?

- Just because something is new, does that mean it has more value?

- Can people become "addicted" to technology or the internet?

- Many of us pick up our phone every time we get bored, lonely, or sad. Is this okay? What are some other things you can do when you feel this way?

ACTIVITIES

Create a Contract
Create a cell phone or social media contract for your child or download one from the internet. (See the "Resources" section below.) Look it over, discuss it with your child, and have your child commit to following the rules laid out in the contract.

Discuss Potential
Talk about the potential for good in all technology. Discuss ways to use phones, tablets, etc. as tools and instruments, not just as a way to pacify or entertain us. Remind your children that they are agents of change! Discuss ways your family can change the world for the better, using technology and good sense.

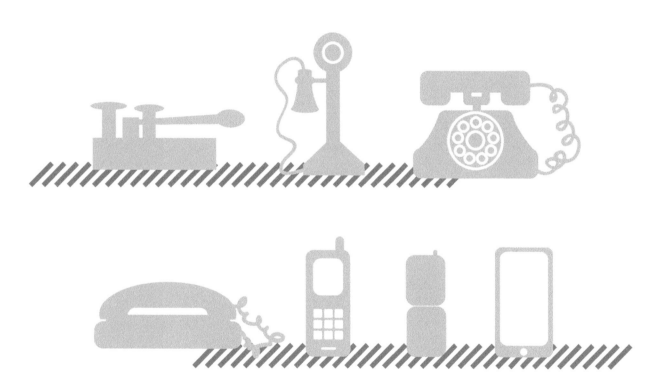

CITATIONS/RESOURCES

Alexander, D. (2017). *Noah's New Phone: A Story About Using Technology for Good.* (J. Webb, M. Warner, and T. Mattsson, eds.). Rising Parent Media.

Bridle, J. (n.d.). The Nightmare Videos of Children's YouTube—and what's Wrong with the Internet Today [Video File]. Retrieved from https://www.ted.com/talks/james_bridle_the_nightmare_videos_of_childrens_youtube_and_what_s_wrong_with_the_internet_today/discussion#t-847196.

Connect Safely. (n.d.). Family Contract for Smartphone Use. Retrieved from https://www.connectsafely.org/family-contract-smartphone-use/.

Lanier, J. (Apr. 2018). How We Need to Remake the Internet [Video File]. Retrieved from https://www.ted.com/talks/jaron_lanier_how_we_need_to_remake_the_internet.

O'Donnell, J. (Aug. 2018). A Sample Cell Phone Contract for Parents and Tweens. Retrieved from https://www.verywellfamily.com/a-sample-cell-phone-contract-for-parents-and-tweens-3288540.

6. ONLINE PORNOGRAPHY

It is natural for kids and adults to be curious, especially about **sex** and our bodies. But it's important for all of us to understand that pornography is not a healthy place to find answers to our questions about sex.

To define **pornography** in a simple way for kids, use the following: Pornography is pictures or videos of people with little or no clothing on. Online pornography usually shows videos of people having sex.

For young kids, it's important to help them know that you understand their curiosity and that you will not shame them for asking questions or talking about issues related to sex. Help them identify possible places they might see porn and teach them a plan for what to do when they encounter porn. (See "RUN Plan" in the activity below.)

For older kids, help them understand the hateful, misogynistic nature of porn, as well as the addictive qualities porn continues to show in various research studies (Your Brain on Porn, n.d.). They should know that the porn industry is actively targeting them (Alexander, 2016) and that you will respond with **compassion** should they start looking at pornography or develop a habit or **addiction**.

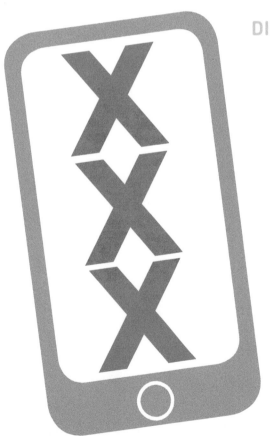

DISCUSSION QUESTIONS

- Why is it natural to be curious about **sex**? What is a healthy way of finding out answers to questions about sex?

- Have you ever seen **pornography**? Where did you first see it? Where are some places one might encounter porn? (the school bus, home computer, summer camp, recess, etc.)

- What is a simple way of telling your friend you don't want to look at something inappropriate on their phone?

- Are there places, online and offline, you can avoid so you don't see pornographic media?

- What can I do as your parent (or trusted adult) to help you feel comfortable talking to me about sex or anything you might have questions about?

♛ Some people seek out pornography when tired, bored, lonely, sad, or stressed out. What do you do when you have these types of feelings?

♛ What are some other activities we can do when we feel bored, lonely, or sad?

ACTIVITY

Teach & Practice the RUN Plan
Talk with your child about what **pornography** is and what they should do if they come across it. Remind them that if they see it, they need to tell you or another trusted adult as soon as possible. (Seeing porn can be very confusing when a child is simultaneously traumatized and aroused at the same time.) Then they need to make a commitment to not seek it out again.

TEACH YOUR KIDS TO:

Recognize what you've seen and get away from it.

Be able to name it when you see it. Decide beforehand how you will get out of the situation.

Understand what you've seen and talk about how it made you feel with a trusted adult.

It's important to tell your parents what you saw. They can help you make sense of the images you have seen and the feelings you may have experienced.

Never seek it out again.

Know where you will be exposed to porn and which friends watch it. Decide what you will say when a friend wants to show you something inappropriate.

DISCUSSION FOR OLDER KIDS & TEENS

Chances are your middle school and high school students have seen a variety of R-rated or pornographic things you have never seen. Ask them to educate you on what kids are talking about and sharing at school or in other activities.

- ♛ What happens when we let porn dictate our ideas about sex instead of creating our own, unique sexuality? How can you create your own ideas about sex with as little media/porn influence as possible?

- ♛ The majority of porn has some form of male domination in it. Why is this a problem?

- ♛ Porn does not portray love, mutual respect, or true **intimacy**. What does real intimacy in a relationship look like?

- ♛ Sexting (trading nudes/sending nudes) has become commonplace among many teenagers despite it being illegal for those under 18 years of age. Do you know about any instances when this was a problem at your school? What happened? How did the kids, parents, teachers, and administrators respond? What would you do if you received a nude picture of one of your friends?

- ♛ What does it mean for us as a society that a majority of teens are watching pornography, where women are portrayed as less-than-human objects to be used, as a means of sex education?

- ♛ Many people think that porn is videotaped prostitution. Do you agree? Do you believe that pornography contributes to human trafficking?

CITATIONS/RESOURCES

Alexander, D., A. Scott, and J. Webb. (2019). *How to Talk to Your Kids About Pornography.* 2nd edition. Rising Parent Media.

Alexander, D. (Feb. 8, 2016). Porn Industry Trends—Where Will They Target Your Children Next? Retrieved from https://educateempowerkids.org/porn-industry-trends-for-2016/.

Alexander, D. (n.d.). Does talking about pornography with your kids "give them ideas"? Retrieved from https://educateempowerkids.org/does-talking-about-pornography-with-your-kids-give-them-ideas/.

Alexander, D. (2018). *Petra's Power to See: A Media Literacy Adventure.* (M. Bergman, ed.). Rising Parent Media.

Your Brain on Porn. (n.d.). Brain Studies on Porn Users & Sex Addicts. Retrieved from https://www.yourbrainonporn.com/relevant-research-and-articles-about-the-studies/brain-studies-on-porn-users-sex-addicts/#brain.

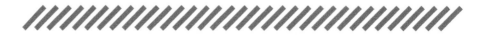

THE WORLD AROUND US

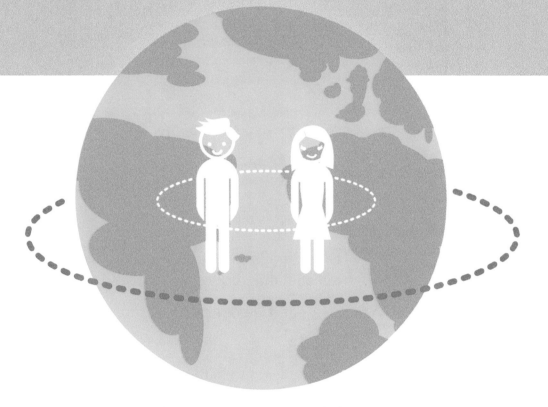

We live in an amazing world that seems to grow a little bit smaller each day as we connect and interact with others. This **globalization** is the result of an increase in technology, particularly over the last 100 years. Although globalization often refers to the spread of economic influence, it also refers to the spread of culture, political and social ideas, and increased cooperation and communication between different people across the world.

Through increased immigration, better education worldwide, numerous global news stories, work participation, social media, and other online experiences there has been an increase in understanding and cooperation between cultures. But we still have a long way to go.

Through these interactions we are able to see the effect of all of our behaviors on the environment and on the health and well-being of other countries and peoples. We can see our errors as well as the advancements we have made. We can observe and learn from the positive and negative attitudes, practices, laws, and traditions of both our culture and other cultures.

7. OUR PLANET AND THE ENVIRONMENT

We live on a beautiful planet, surrounded by natural resources and living things that depend on us for their survival. As parents, we need to teach our kids to appreciate the world around them. We also need to teach them that the choices they make will have an effect on the environment–now and in the future.

Unfortunately, **environmental issues** have also taken on a heavily political flavor in today's world. As a result, we are constantly bombarded with media messages about the environment that look and sound a lot like *advertising,* and people in power use these ideas as a source of contention. In our families, we can do better! We can rise above the media madness and concentrate on small choices that we make every day.

Take time to talk with your children about environmental issues like pollution, recycling, and climate change to empower them when they encounter these ideas in the world.

DISCUSSION QUESTIONS

- What is recycling? Is it better to use a trash service or a recycling service?

- Do we have a recycling service in our area? Do we recycle at our house? Why or why not?

- What happens to our trash after the truck comes to pick it up?

- What is littering? What happens if we don't pick up litter?

- What is a **carbon footprint**?

- What are some things we already do to help the environment?

- What are some things we can do better when it comes to the environment?

- What happens to the waste after we flush the toilet?

- Where does the water in our faucet come from? Why does this matter?

- What is **global warming**? Is global warming real?

- Why are people on the news always arguing about the environment?

- Is there really a hole in the ozone layer? What does that mean? How did it get there?

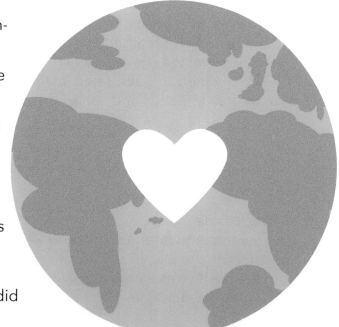

- What kinds of energy produce pollution? What are some forms of alternative energy? How does water/air/land become polluted?

- Why are people so upset about the rainforests disappearing?

- Do trees really produce the oxygen we need to breathe? What would happen if there were no more trees on our planet?

ACTIVITIES

Outdoor Preparation
Pretend you are going on a family picnic, hike, or campout. What are some choices you would make that could help protect the environment?

Discover Decomposition
Decomposition is the breakdown of matter by bacteria and fungi. It changes the composition of the materials into something more natural, like dirt (Decomposition, n.d.). How long do you think it would take for these items to decompose: newspaper, orange peel, leaves, aluminum cans, plastic bottle, glass bottle, styrofoam cup. Do a search for "estimated decomposition rates" online to find out!

Trash Patrol!
As a family, go on a walk and pick up trash in your neighborhood.

DISCUSSION FOR OLDER KIDS & TEENS

Did you know that there is a giant pile of plastic and trash floating in the Pacific Ocean, between California and Hawaii? It's called the "Great Pacific Garbage Patch" and scientists say it is now three times the size of France and growing at an exponential rate. How do you think this affects the plants and animals in our beautiful ocean? If the Garbage Patch continues to grow at this alarming rate, what do you think will happen? Can you think of any possible solutions to this problem?

CITATIONS/RESOURCES

ABC News. (2018). 'Great Pacific Garbage Patch' is Massive Floating Island of Plastic, Now 3 Times the Size of France. Retrieved from https://abcnews.go.com/International/great-pacific-garbage-patch-massive-floating-island-plastic/story?id=53962147.

Decomposition. (n.d.). U.S. Environmental Protection Agency. Retrieved from http://www.ecologydictionary.org/EPA-Glossary-of-Climate-Change-Terms/.

8. RACISM AND TOLERANCE

Today's world is a lot smaller than it used to be! Over the past 100 years, we have gained the ability to cross more borders and meet more people than ever before—allowing us to accept and embrace the beautiful diversity of the cultures and races that surround us.

Our children, who are now growing up in a digital age, truly are global citizens. As we teach them to explore their world, it is crucial that we teach them to do so with an open mind. In an image-based culture that entices us to make judgements at a glance, we must teach them to see past the outside appearance, and to look deeper. We can start at home by modeling virtues like kindness and **tolerance** and rejecting attitudes that project hate, fear, and **racism** toward others.

However, it's not enough to just talk about racism. Our subtle attitudes and small actions are being watched and absorbed by our children. We may not even be aware that we are conveying our ideas about race through our behaviors, but we are (Hagerman, 2018)! Our conversations definitely matter, but so does everything else we do. As we think critically about race and tolerance, reexamine our behaviors, and teach our children to do the same, we can help create a better world.

- -

DISCUSSION QUESTIONS

- Why are people different from each other? What would it be like if we were all the same?

- Does skin color really matter?

- Do you have any friends who belong to different religions, races, or cultures than you do? What do you think about that?

- Why do women in some cultures cover their heads with scarves?

- If someone doesn't speak English, does that mean they are not intelligent?

- What is **racism**?

- Why is it difficult for many people to talk about race?

- What is **implicit bias**?

- What are some times in history (and now) when racism became a problem?

- Can you think of any historical connections between racism and slavery? Why is this significant?

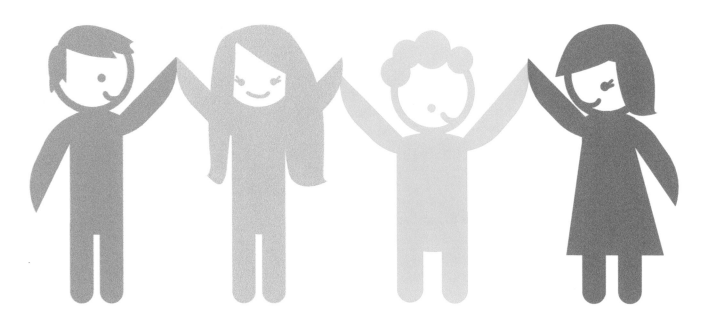

- Can you think of any historical (or present-day) examples of racism that led to war?

- Have you seen any examples of hate or racism in school or in our neighborhood?

- Is there a connection between hate, racism, fear, and violence?

- Can racism lead to **bullying**?

- What are some solutions to racism?

- What is the opposite of racism?

- How would the world be different if there were no racism?

- What are some specific ways we can show **tolerance** toward people who are different than us at school? in our community? online/on social media?

- What is **tolerance**? How can we be more tolerant and kind to people of all cultures?

- People from different countries eat different food, wear different clothes, and have different ideas and customs. Why is that something we can appreciate and enjoy?

- What are some different cultures that you would like to learn about?

ACTIVITIES

I Have a Dream
Look up the transcript from the "I Have a Dream" speech by Martin Luther King, Jr. Do some research about the time period when it was given. What is this speech about? What do these words mean to you? Why was this speech so important?

New Kid
Imagine that a new boy moved into your school. He doesn't speak English, and he wears clothes that are different from you and your friends. He sits alone at lunch and eats food that seems strange to you. He has a name that many people can't pronounce. No one picks him for teams in gym class. Some of the other kids start making fun of him—pointing and teasing every day when he passes in the hallway. What would you do? What if you moved to a different country and the situation were reversed (you were the new kid)? How would you feel?

DISCUSSION FOR OLDER KIDS & TEENS

Racism is believed by many to be an ideology that originated from European scientists in the 17th century during the Atlantic slave trade. It is said they invented it in order to differentiate themselves from those with different skin colors and darker features, creating a racial hierarchy that continues to this day. It would simply be incorrect to deny that the history of racism has been (and continues to be) one of white supremacy as the label "white" has always been an indication of superiority (Whitaker, 2017). Do you agree with this assessment? Where could you find out more information about the history of racism and how to uproot it?

CITATIONS/RESOURCES

Hagerman, M. A. (Sep. 4, 2018). Why White Parents Can't Just Talk to Their Kids About Racism. Retrieved from http://time.com/5362786/talking-racism-with-white-kids-not-enough/.

Tolerance, s.v. Merriam-Webster Online. Retrieved from https://www.merriam-webster.com/dictionary/tolerance.

Whitaker, S. (Feb. 19, 2017). Dear White People, Your "Dictionary Definition" of Racism is Wrong. Retrieved from http://affinitymagazine.us/2017/02/19/dear-white-people-your-dictionary-definition-of-racism-is-wrong/.

9. FEMINISM

Like it or not, throughout history (and in many cultures) females have often been viewed as the lesser or "weaker" gender. As a result, women and girls have been denied the same opportunities as men when it comes to education, politics, or even the right to live—simply because they are female. Essentially, **feminism** is the reaction to this philosophy. It is the umbrella term that describes all women and men who stand up and say, "No way! Women are not weaker! They are just as strong, intelligent, and capable as the men!" Feminists are people who support this philosophy. They advocate for equal rights between men and women and often rally together to fight for the cause.

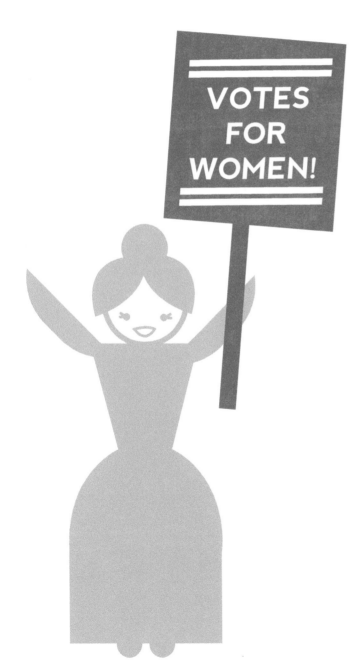

Over the years, feminists have taken on several causes. Women in the United States and the United Kingdom fought for their right to vote and own property in the early 1900s. This era was known as the suffrage movement or the "first wave" of feminism.

During the 1960s through the 1980s, the "second wave" of the feminist movement began focusing on issues related to sexuality and reproduction that included the abortion debate. Other issues facing modern feminism include equal pay, stereotypes in the media, and violence against women (Cosslett, 2013).

Although some may generalize all feminists as "man-haters" who think that women should rule the world and disenfranchise all men, this is a **stereotype**.

However, because much of "second wave" feminism focused on equality this has led to many current feminist philosophies to reject the gender binary today. "Gender binary" is the classification of sex and gender into only two options as male and female, masculine and feminine. Because of this, there has been a movement to broaden the idea of sexuality and sexual expression and to reject the idea of purely masculine and feminine roles as well as the rejection of sexual assignment of being either male or female. As a result, feminism has paved the way for much of the LGBTQI movement to become mainstream.

In a world where feminism is part of often contentious political debates and regularly featured in the media, our kids are destined to be surrounded by messages about these issues and philosophies, especially since feminism is now linked to the sexual and transgender movement that is affecting many children and families today. As parents, we can educate them about feminism and gender roles, allowing them to navigate our culture with confidence.

DISCUSSION QUESTIONS

- What is **feminism**? Is there only one definition of feminism?

- What is a feminist? Is there only one way to be a feminist? Who can be a feminist? What does feminism mean to you?

- Is feminism a good thing or a bad thing?

- Do you think women should have the same rights as men? Do you think women in other countries should have the same rights as men? Why or why not?

- Do you think women should be the *same* as men? Why or why not?

- Who do you think is smarter: men or women? Who do you think is stronger: men or women? Why? Is it possible that men can be strong in their own way, and that women can be strong in their own way?

- What kinds of things affect the way you think about women? Media? Friends? What else?

- What is gender? What are gender roles?

- What are the major issues that face women today here and in other countries?

- Do you think women and men should unite to fight for their rights? Do you think it's important for women and men to fight for their rights in other countries?

- What are some victories won by feminists throughout history? How have these victories affected your life?

👑 Do you consider yourself to be a feminist? Why or why not?

👑 Do you know anyone who considers herself/himself to be a feminist?

ACTIVITY AND DISCUSSION FOR OLDER KIDS & TEENS

Title IX
Title IX is a law that prevents gender discrimination in sports programs at schools that receive federal funding. (See Title IX and Sex Discrimination below for more information.) Do an internet search for news articles about sports programs at schools and universities that might have been affected by this law. After reading through these articles, what did you learn? How do you feel about Title IX?

Gender Stereotypes
Think about the last movie or TV show you watched. Were there any gender stereotypes? A gender **stereotype** teaches us unspoken rules that males and females are supposed to follow. For example: "men have big muscles and women wear makeup" or "boys wear blue and girls wear pink" or "mothers are caring and fathers protect their families." Where did these rules come from? Who made them? Are these ideas healthy or unhealthy for society? (Hint: The answer might be different for each stereotype.) Did you realize there were stereotypes in the show you were watching? We need to be careful about media. Often, we are absorbing lessons about society without even realizing it!

Types of Feminism
There are several belief systems within the feminist movement. Take a few minutes— or more—to find out about Radical Feminism, Liberal Feminism, Maternal Feminism, EcoFeminism, and others.

CITATIONS/RESOURCES

Cosslett, R. & H. Baxter. (2013). The Five Main Issues Facing Modern Feminism. Retrieved from https://www.new-statesman.com/v-spot/2013/05/five-main-issues-facing-modern-feminism.

Eagle, A. (2003). Learn Where You Fit In Feminist Spectrum: A New Study Shows Women Combine Features Of Femininity, Masculinity And Feminist Ideals. Retrieved from http://articles.orlandosentinel.com/2003-01-20/news/0301190005_1_femininity-masculinity-feminist-ideals.

Office for Civil Rights. (2015). Title IX and Sex Discrimination. Retrieved from https://www2.ed.gov/about/offices/list/ocr/docs/tix_dis.html.

ADDITIONAL RESOURCE

Big Ocean Women is an international, interfaith organization that celebrates maternal feminism, which recognizes and honors mothers as a powerful force in society. https://www.bigoceanwomen.org/about-us/our-beliefs/

10. SOCIAL CLASSES: RICH AND POOR

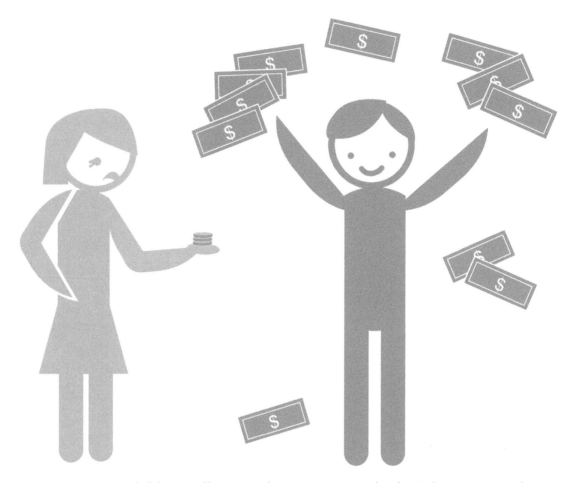

At some point, your children will notice that some people don't have as much money as others, and they likely will have some questions about it. Kids talk. They notice who has the nicest sneakers, the newest phone, or the best name brands on clothes. They whisper about the kid who has an old hand-me-down backpack and gossip about whose parents seem to give their kids money whenever they want.

So how will our kids act in these situations? Will they be the ones pointing a finger? Will they turn up their nose to a beggar on the street? Or will they have a compassionate heart? And what does **compassion** look like—a handout, a willingness to sit and visit, a donation of time or resources to a charity? As parents, it's our job to start these kinds of conversations at home and set an example with our actions. We have a chance to shape our children's attitudes right from the start. With a little direction, we can teach our kids to have an educated heart when it comes to **social classes**.

As our kids get older, they will notice friends or members of the community who work just as hard as you do, but don't have as nice of clothes or as big of a house. They may notice that *your* family isn't able to go on big vacations like the Jones family. Soon they will pick up on the fact that the United States is an incredibly wealthy country compared to many other countries. They will see that there are not as many minorities as white people in certain professions. They will hear the word "privilege." Be prepared to talk about these issues.

When talking about poverty or wealth, speak in concrete terms: some people have just what they need, some people have more than they need and some people, unfortunately, don't have what they need. Talk about our relationship with money. Discuss the fact that although we live in a wealthy country our citizens are not any happier than those living in poorer countries.

DISCUSSION QUESTIONS

- Can money make people happy?

- Does having a nice car make one person better than another?

- Does money make people smarter?

- Why are people so focused on making more money?

- What if money didn't exist? How would the world be different?

- Why are some people rich and other people poor?

- There are many **prejudices** people have toward poor people. What are some of these?

- Why do some people think that if someone is poor then they must be lazy or dumb?

- Why are some people homeless?

- Why do some people stand on the street begging for money?

- Why are there "rich" parts of a city and "poor" parts of a city?

- Why is it important to have a job?

- Does having a job mean that we can buy anything we want?

- If I work hard can I have any job I want or make as much money as I want?

- There are poor and hungry people in every country. Why is that, when some countries like the United States are very wealthy?

- How can we be more empathetic to people around us who have less than we do?

- How can you be kind to other kids at school who don't have as much as you?

- What can we do to help others in financial need?

ACTIVITIES

Volunteer Together
Locate a homeless shelter or soup kitchen in your area, and find out if you and your family can do some service there. After you go, reflect on the experience together. Talk about the people there. What if you were in their shoes? How would you feel?

Welcome Refugees
Talk to a local refugee center. Find out what their real needs are for people immigrating to our country with no more than a backpack of items or just the clothes on their back. With your kids, determine how you can be helpful. Is it collecting and delivering furniture or toiletries? Make a plan and follow through together.

DISCUSSION FOR OLDER KIDS & TEENS

In 1848, Karl Marx published *The Communist Manifesto*. Marx believed in a socialist state where everyone was equal—no rich and no poor. Many people throughout history have explored alternatives to **capitalism**. Some of those other systems, like the Soviet Union, were authoritarian and repressive. Other approaches, such as worker-owned co-operative businesses, have been successful. Do some research on countries and small communities who have tried alternatives to capitalism. Can people eliminate **social classes**? What could unsuccessful attempts like the Soviet Union have done differently? Where do you see successful alternatives to capitalism?

CITATIONS/RESOURCES

Feuer, L. & D. McLellan. (Jan. 21, 2019). Karl Marx: German Philosopher. Retrieved from https://www.britannica.com/biography/Karl-Marx.

Morin, A. (Feb. 14, 2018.). How to Talk to Kids About Poverty. Retrieved from https://www.verywellfamily.com/how-to-talk-to-kids-about-poverty-4142890.

Simons, S. (Jun. 27, 2018). How to Talk to Kids About Rich People. Retrieved from https://www.fatherly.com/love-money/how-to-talk-to-kids-about-rich-people/.

11. TERRORISM, WAR, AND PEACE

Our world is constantly in motion. Political unrest across international borders, spontaneous bombings, and flags flying at half-mast are just part of the deal. From a child's perspective, these events can seem scary and unsettling. Instead of glossing over these issues or pretending the news doesn't exist, we can look for ways to address these topics with our kids. It's okay to acknowledge the fact that we flow through different times of war and peace. Remind your kids that your home is a safe place, and that you have their backs. This will help them feel more secure in the world around them.

It can be difficult to talk not only about **terrorism** but also about U.S. leaders who have used war and violence to control other countries. How do you explain something that we don't quite understand? When these events happen, acknowledge your own feelings and model healthy coping skills for your kids. Listen to your kids' worries. Reassure them and emphasize that while there are some bad people in the world, there are many, many more good people.

DISCUSSION QUESTIONS

- What are some significant acts of terrorism that have taken place during your lifetime?

- For parents: Were you alive during the September 11th terrorist attacks on the U.S.? If so, where were you? What do you remember about that day?

- Why does **terrorism** exist in our world?

- Why do you think people join terrorist organizations?

- How would you feel if someone asked you to join a terrorist organization?

- What kind of people do you think terrorist organizations look for when they are recruiting new members?

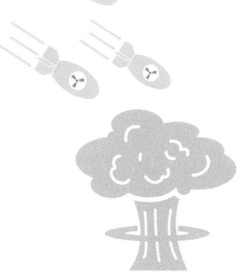

- Have any of our family members fought in the military? If so, what are some of the stories they brought home?

- Did any of our family members fight in World War II, Korea, or Vietnam? How did these wars affect our family?

♕ What does war look like?

♕ How has war changed in the past 100 years?

♕ How has technology changed the way war looks?

♕ Why do some countries live in peace, while others have turmoil?

♕ Are there any wars going on in the world right now?

♕ Would you ever want to fight in a war? Why or why not?

♕ Are their good and just reasons for a country to go to war?

♕ Why is peace between countries important?

♕ Is there anything you can do to stop a war?

DISCUSSION FOR OLDER KIDS & TEENS

It has been argued that if people who are recruited by terrorist groups had jobs and enough food to eat that they would not want to be terrorists. What do you think?

Some terrorist organizations, like ISIS, actively recruit kids online—especially through social media channels. What would you do if you encountered a recruiter like this online?

CITATIONS/RESOURCES

Bouzar, D. and C. R. Flynn. (Sep. 5, 2017). ISIS Recruiting: It's Not (Just) Ideological. Retrieved from https://www.fpri.org/article/2017/09/isis-recruiting-not-just-ideological/.

Steinberg, B. (Nov. 2, 2017). ABC News Will Air Diane Sawyer ISIS Investigation on Friday's '20/20'. Retrieved from https://variety.com/2017/tv/news/diane-sawyer-2020-isis-investigation-1202605261/.

12. HEALTH, DISEASE, AND PREVENTION

With modern technology and nonstop news, we are more aware of sickness, disease, new medicines, and health problems than ever before. This overload of information can be overwhelming—and even a little scary—for our children.

On the flip side, our culture makes promises about cures and health and fitness that seem too good to be true. And many of them are! Skinny, muscular models gloss the pages of magazines and billboards. Ads hint at eternal youth and perfect health if we just purchase that miracle diet, powerful pill or powder, or countless other products.

What is true? What isn't? What should we believe about our bodies? When it comes to health and disease, we have a responsibility to sort through the madness and figure it out with our kids!

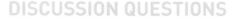

DISCUSSION QUESTIONS

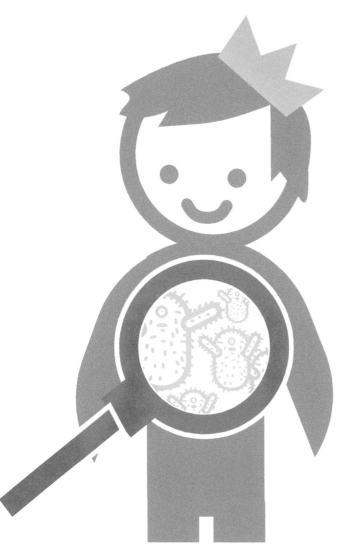

- What does it mean to be healthy? What are some things that healthy people do?

- What does a healthy body look like? Is there only one healthy body type?

- Is "skinny" the same thing as "healthy"?

- How do you feel about your body? What are some things you are grateful your body can do?

- What are some things you do to keep your body healthy?

- What is the difference between healthy food and unhealthy food?

- What is "junk food"? What are some examples? Is it ok to eat this kind of food? Why or why not?

- Why do we have doctors?

- How does medication work? Why do we need medication?

- What is preventive medicine? Do we spend more time and money treating disease, or preventing it? Why or why not?

- Why do we get sick? What is an immune system? How does it work?

- What are some ways that people spread germs? What are some easy ways to help stop the spread of germs during cold and flu season?

- What is an "invisible disease"? What does that term mean? What is an example of an invisible disease?

- Heart disease is the leading cause of death in the United States. What is heart disease? What are some good ways to help prevent it?

- What are some habits that contribute to a healthy lifestyle and prevent other diseases? What are some unhealthy habits?

- What kinds of diseases are preventable? What kinds of diseases cannot be prevented? Do all diseases have a cure?

- How would things in our family be different if one of our family members got very sick?

- What is a chronic illness?

- What is mental illness?

- Why do people smoke?

- What are some illegal substances? Why are they illegal? What kinds of effects do they have on the body?

- Have you ever had surgery? What was it like?

- Why do people have surgery?

- What kinds of messages does the media teach us about health?

- What are some reliable sources to find out about health and disease?

ACTIVITY

Media Messages about Food
Teach your kids to question the messages they are receiving about health through the media. Find an ad that shows happy children eating candy or junk food. Show the ad to your child, and then reflect on it together. Ask them: What is this ad really saying? Does this mean that kids are only really happy when they eat this specific brand of food or candy? Are we healthy and happy when we eat junk food?

DISCUSSION FOR OLDER KIDS & TEENS

What is "big pharma"? Why do people on the news argue about this topic?

Many "health" magazines actually feature sexualized images and even airbrushed photos of popular athletes that objectify these individuals and make them look more muscular or skinnier than they really are. Is this honest? Is it healthy? How does this affect our cultural attitudes toward health and fitness?

CITATIONS/RESOURCES

Andrews, C. and A. Scott (n.d.). Bodily Integrity: Teaching Your Child to Make the Best Choices for His or Her Body. Retrieved from https://educateempowerkids.org/bodily-integrity.

Alexander, D. (2018). *Petra's Power to See: A Media Literacy Adventure.* (M. Bergman, ed.). Rising Parent Media.

Alexander, D. and K. Roberts. (2017). *Messages About Me: Sydney's Story: A Girl's Journey to Healthy Body Image.* (J. Webb, ed.). Rising Parent Media.

Alexander, D. and K. Roberts. (2017). *Messages About Me: Wade's Story: A Boy's Quest for Healthy Body Image.* Rising Parent Media.

Krause, E. (n.d.) Four Ways to Instill a Healthy Body Image in Your Children. Retrieved from https://educateempowerkids.org/four-ways-instill-healthy-body-image-children.

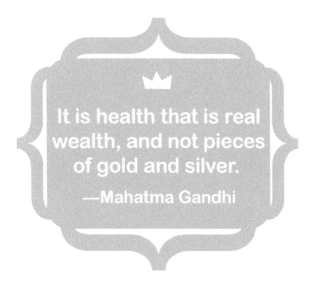

It is health that is real wealth, and not pieces of gold and silver.
—Mahatma Gandhi

13. GIVING AND SERVING

As the years pass and our culture becomes more self-centered, it is so important to teach our kids to think about others. But as the saying goes, "actions speak louder than words." We can't just tell our kids to be kind. We need to *show* them. As parents, we can set the example and then work together, serving others as a family.

Remember, our balance of *giving* versus *receiving* depends largely on what we learn at a young age. Teach your kids that giving and serving is more than just grand gestures at Christmastime. It can be small and simple everyday actions.

Let your kids know that serving isn't usually easy or convenient. It may involve work, but it should not require a physical or tangible reward. We don't serve and give so that we can get a treat, brag about it, or get attention. We give because it is the right thing to do.

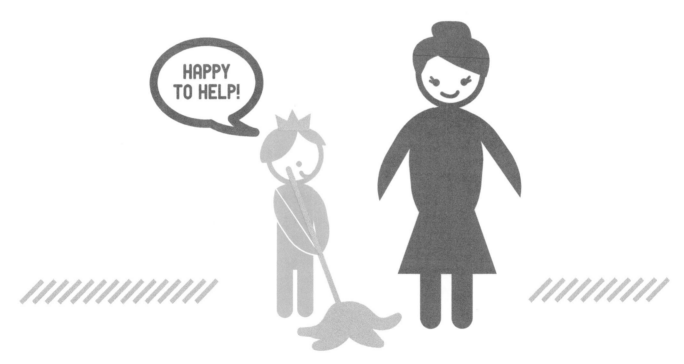

DISCUSSION QUESTIONS

- Winston Churchill said, "We make a living by what we get, but we make a life by what we give." What does this mean?

- How can we help someone who doesn't have enough food to eat? Clothes to wear? A warm place to sleep?

- Can we find a way to give our extra toys or other items to needy children?

- When was the last time you called your grandma or grandpa on the phone?

- Do we have any lonely neighbors that might like a visit or a plate of cookies?

- Where is the nearest homeless shelter? What do you think it would be like to live there?

- What do you think it is like living in a nursing home? Do you think we could find some time to visit a nursing home and cheer up the people who live there?

- What are some ways that you can serve members of your family? What are some ways that you can serve your friends?

- What are some of your talents? How can you use your talents to help others?

- How do you feel when you serve others?

- Do we have to tell someone when we do something nice for them? Or can we do it in secret?

- Do you have any ideas about how to serve others in your community?

- Do we always have to do something big in order to serve others? Or can we do little things too?

- Can you think of some small ways to serve your friends and neighbors?

ACTIVITIES

Give Your Time
Find a way for your family to volunteer. Visit a homeless shelter, food bank, women's shelter, refugee center, or soup kitchen. Almost all of these places are underfunded and don't have enough resources or people to fill all the needs that are asked of them. Donate a few hours of your time to help the people there. Afterward, reflect on the experience with your family.

Other Ways to Give of Your Time or Resources
Take treats to a neighbor, volunteer at a local library, help out at an animal shelter, ask your pastor or other church leaders if there is a family in your congregation that has a need, mow your neighbor's yard, write a letter to a faraway relative, visit people at a nursing home, babysit for free, or reach out to your local United Way and find a project you can participate in.

CITATIONS/RESOURCES

King, K. (n.d.). 'Tis the Season to Serve: Simple Online Ways Our Families Can Serve. Retrieved from https://educate-empowerkids.org/tis-season-serve-simple-online-ways-families-can-serve.

King, K. and M. Bergman. (n.d.). Creating Purpose in Summertime: Simple Online Ways to Serve. Retrieved from https://educateempowerkids.org/creating-purpose-summertime-simple-online-ways-serve.

RELATIONSHIPS

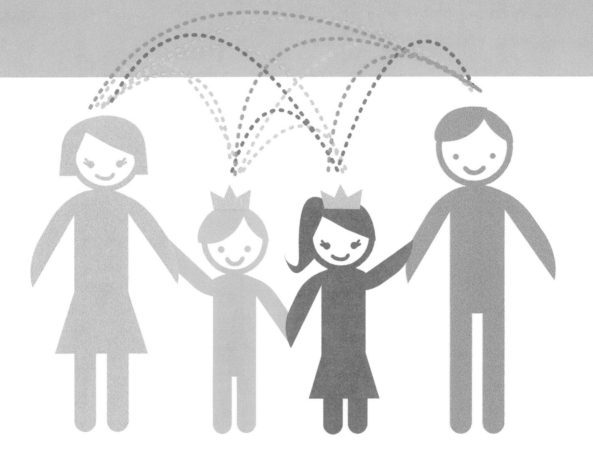

Love, family relationships, friendships, acquaintances, romantic relationships—these are some of the most wonderful (and the most difficult) experiences of our lives. They give us purpose, comfort, fulfillment, **joy**, laughter, and more. They also bring us heartache, sadness, frustration, and rejection. Through the good and the bad, relationships are what make life worth living.

And just like our bodies require nutritious food, rest, and exercise, relationships need positive communication, **empathy**, and kindness to be healthy. Teaching our kids how to build healthy relationships will enable them to recognize when a relationship is *unhealthy*, build healthy relationships, and allow them to help others to foster healthy relationships. This is critical, especially as strong, healthy relationships are the foundation of society.

14. GETTING ALONG AND STANDING UP FOR OTHERS

Relationships are part of everyone's daily lives. Some of these relationships are serious or familial. Some relationships are short-lived or passing. We don't have to "like" or enjoy everyone around us, but we do need to get along. Usually getting along is the first step in building a deep, meaningful relationship. These meaningful relationships are often built upon mutual respect, open communication, and unselfishness by both people involved.

The opposite of getting along is **bullying**, which has changed over the years. Once viewed as "kids being kids" or as something that will work itself out, bullying has become a huge social problem that can no longer be dismissed or ignored.

In particular, **cyberbullying** has rewritten the rules of bullying in sneaky, sinister ways. It's easier to dehumanize a victim when you're hiding behind a screen or a text. Also, unlike the schoolyard bully of the past who remained at school, the cyberbully follows our children wherever they go, day and night. With the addition of social media and mass texting, cyberbullies are provided with a platform to humiliate their victims on an enormous scale, resulting in hopelessness and in serious cases, even suicide (McKenna, n.d.).

In a world like this, we need to be proactive. When we see a problem or when someone is bullying, we need to stand up for ourselves and others. We need to ask for help when we encounter a bullying situation—whether in person or online. As parents, we need to teach our kids that their actions have great power and that they can have a lasting effect on everyone around them.

DISCUSSION QUESTIONS

- What is meant by the famous quote from John Donne, "No man is an island"?

- Why do people need other people?

- There are people of different cultures, races, and **religions** all over the world. Why is it so important for us to get along?

- What are some of the consequences of *not* getting along?

- What are the benefits of getting along with others?

- What makes someone a good friend? How do they treat you?

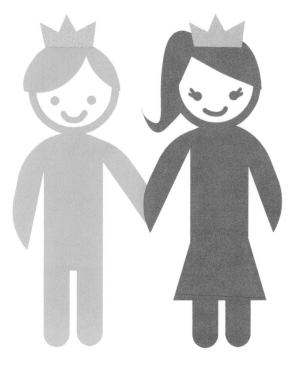

- Do you treat your family members as well as you treat your friends?

- Why is it sometimes difficult to get along with the people we live with?

- Why is it sometimes hard to get along with various kids at school?

- How could you be a better friend? What do you look for in a friend?

- How can you show respect to people you don't agree with?

- Can you think of a time you had a problem with someone and you worked it out? How did you feel afterward?

- What is a bully?

- What is a victim?

- What is **cyberbullying**?

- What is the difference between someone who is being annoying and rude and someone who is really bullying?

- What can you do if you see someone being bullied?

- What are some ways you can stand up to a bully who is picking on you?

- -

- If a bully is hurting you, should you hurt them back?

- If you are being bullied at school, should you tell the teacher?

- What should you do if you see a bunch of kids gang up on one person? If your friends are making fun of someone who seems different than everyone else, should you join in?

- What are some reasons that bullies might pick on other kids?

- Are bullies bad kids?

- What are some ways kids and adults bully each other online, through texting and social media?

👑 Is it possible to be bullied by someone who is your friend?

👑 Is it possible for someone to be both a victim and a bully?

👑 What can you do to make sure you are not bullying others?

ACTIVITIES

To Have a Good Friend, You Need to Be One
Write the following phrases on slips of paper. Have family or class members take turns picking a slip out of a hat or bowl. Ask the person who has pulled out the slip to read the slip of paper and then tell why this behavior is that of a good friend or not.

Phrases to write:

> Be yourself.
> Include someone who is feeling left out.
> Get to know others by asking questions and listening.
> Say good things about others.
> Show interest in what others are doing.
> Help others.
> Invite others to do something with you.
> Lie about others so you will seem to be the only worthwhile friend to have.
> Buy friendship by giving treats and expensive gifts.
> Be fake or give false praise.
> Threaten to desert your friend if he/she won't agree with you.
> Be rude to people you don't like.

Dealbreakers
Help your child role-play things in a friendship that are unacceptable to them or "deal-breakers" (for example, lying, stealing, publicly embarrassing you, etc.). Help your child understand that sometimes friendships don't work out. Ask your child, "How would you decide if you should or should not be friends with someone anymore?" and "How will you decide if something should be forgiven?"

Online Bullying
Many anonymous apps and social media outlets are used for bullying. What apps and social media are popular at your school?

Embarrassing Photo
You are checking your text messages and receive an embarrassing photo of a girl you don't know. After talking to your friends, you find out the girl in the photo goes to your school, and that all your friends received the embarrassing photo too. In fact, it turns out that pretty much everyone in the school received the photo. What should you do? How would you feel if you were the person in the photo?

CITATIONS/RESOURCES

Alexander, D., et. al. (2016). *30 Days to a Stronger Child*. Rising Parent Media.

Alexander, D. (2017). *Noah's New Phone: A Story About Using Technology for Good*. (J. Webb, M. Warner, and T. Mattsson, eds.). Rising Parent Media.

Cagle, C. (n.d.) Back-to-school anti-bullying strategies. Retrieved from https://educateempowerkids.org/back-school-anti-bullying-strategies.

Church Jesus Christ of Latter-day Saints. (n.d.). Retrieved from https://www.lds.org/manual/family-home-evening-resource-book?lang=eng.

Educate and Empower Kids. (2018). Lesson: How to Create Healthy Relationships. Retrieved from https://educateempowerkids.org/wp-content/uploads/2018/06/Healthy-Relationships-Lesson-Plan.pdf.

Educate and Empower Kids. (n.d.) Lesson: Kindness: Online, Face to Face, and Everywhere. Retrieved from https://educateempowerkids.org/wp-content/uploads/2018/03/Kindness-Lesson-Plan.pdf.

Gordon, S. (n.d.). 6 Types of Bullying Parents Should Know About. Retrieved from https://www.verywellfamily.com/types-of-bullying-parents-should-know-about-4153882.

Loyd, K. (n.d.) Four Simple Ways to Strengthen Your Relationship with Your Child this Year. Retrieved from https://educateempowerkids.org/four-ways-strengthen-relationship-child-year.

McKenna, C. (n.d.). Snapchat Suicide: Is Social Media Killing Our Kids? Retrieved from https://protectyoungeyes.com/snapchat-suicide-social-media-killing-our-kids/.

Steyskal-Rondeau, M. (n.d.) How to Raise a Bully. Retrieved from https://educateempowerkids.org/how-to-raise-a-bully.

Steyskal-Rondeau, M. (n.d.). Giving a Voice to Bullying Victims. Retrieved from https://educateempowerkids.org/giving-a-voice-to-bullying-victims/.

ADDITIONAL RESOURCES

Because of You is a movement that encourages teens to reflect on the power of their words and actions, and to consider the effects they can have on others. https://becauseofyou.org

The Cybersmile Foundation helps reduce cyberbullying through public awareness campaigns, the promotion of positive digital citizenship, and professional support for victims and their families. https://www.cybersmile.org/who-we-are

The National Center for Bullying Prevention provides tools for parents, students and teachers, and recognizes bullying as a serious community issue. https://www.pacer.org/bullying/

STOMP Out Bullying works to deter bullying in schools, online, and in communities all throughout the country. https://stompoutbullying.org/

The Stop Bullying Campaign by Cartoon Network encourages kids to speak up through PSA's inspired by real kids' stories. https://www.cartoonnetwork.com/stop-bullying/index.html

15. COMPASSION AND EMPATHY

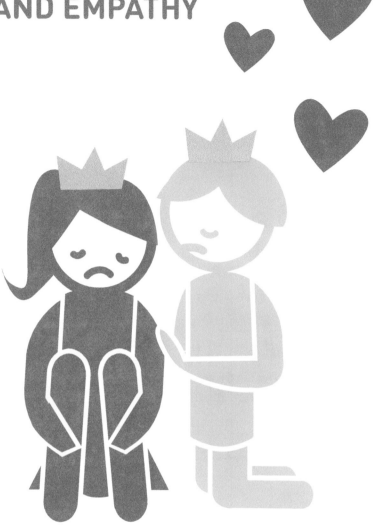

Empathy and **compassion** are critical components in developing emotional intelligence. We develop these skills as we become aware of other people's feelings, needs, and concerns. Empathy is important because it helps us to understand how others are feeling and how our actions might impact them. It's important for building relationships with friends and family. The best way to teach empathy to our kids is to model it, especially for our kids' concerns, feelings, and perceptions.

Experts have become increasingly concerned that too much screen time may be causing a decline in empathy because we are replacing the role of real live friends with virtual ones (Swanbrow, 2010). If we are to teach our kids to have empathy for others or feel compassion then we must exemplify these traits in our words and our actions.

Empathy is often confused with sympathy; however, they are not the same thing. Sympathy is a feeling of pity and sorrow for someone else's misfortune. Empathy goes beyond pity and focuses on having a personal understanding and sharing emotions with someone. Compassion is the added feeling of having empathy and includes the desire to help.

DISCUSSION QUESTIONS

- What is the difference between **empathy** and **compassion**?

- What does it mean to share someone's emotions?

- Can you think of a time when you were experiencing a strong emotion and someone helped you? What did the person do to support you? How did the support you received make you feel towards the other person?

- How can you help others when they are having an emotional challenge?

- How can helping people manage their emotions build a strong friendship network, family, and community?

- When you see other people who are sad or afraid how does it make you feel? Can you help them? How?

- How does it make you feel when someone gives you a hug when you are sad?

- How does it make you feel when others listen to you and show they understand after you've had a bad day?

- When someone is sad, what can you say to them to help them feel better?

- What can you do to help others feel better?

ACTIVITIES

The "What if" Game
Set up some scenarios by asking your child "What if" questions, like the samples below. In each scenario, have them tell you how they think the person would feel and then give you examples of ways they might be able to help.

- What if you saw someone get pushed down on the playground? How do you think they would feel? What could you do to help them?

- What if your friend won their soccer championship? How do you think they would feel? How could you share in their emotion with them?

- What if your friend's pet died? How do you think they would feel? What could you do to help them?

- What if your friend couldn't find their phone or tablet? How do you think they would feel? What could you do to help them?

Challenge

Ask your child to think of someone they know who is sad, lonely, or isolated, and decide how they can show they care for that person. Brainstorm ideas together. Remind them to consider the person's situation and take that into account. For example, your child could choose to write a letter, bake cookies, or simply smile at a clerk in the grocery store. Assist your child with the follow-through and help them to recognize how paying attention to their natural **empathy** strengthens their relationship with others.

CITATIONS/RESOURCES

Alexander, D., et. al. (2016). *30 Days to a Stronger Child.* Rising Parent Media.

Benson, M. (n.d.). Teach More than "Charity" this Season, Teach Your Kids Empathy! Retrieved from https://educate-empowerkids.org/teach-charity-season-teach-kids-empathy/.

Educate and Empower Kids. (Sep. 7, 2016). Five Ways to Teach Your Child Empathy. Retrieved from https://educate-empowerkids.org/five-ways-teach-child-empathy/.

Swanbrow, D. (May 27, 2010). Empathy: College Students Don't Have as Much as They Used To. Retrieved from https://news.umich.edu/empathy-college-students-don-t-have-as-much-as-they-used-to/.

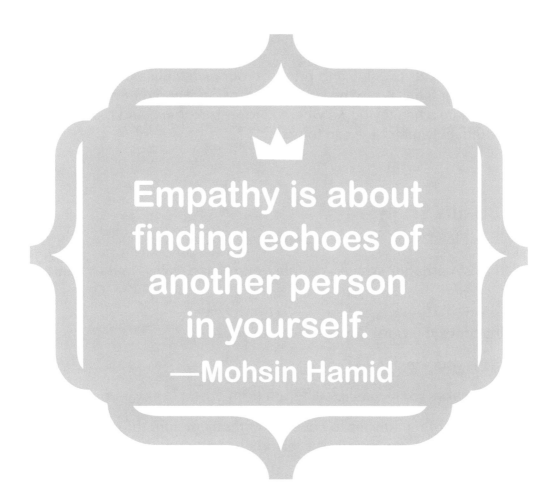

Empathy is about finding echoes of another person in yourself.
—Mohsin Hamid

16. FAMILY, LOVE, MARRIAGE, DIVORCE, AND EVERYTHING IN BETWEEN

Every family is different and special in its own way. Whether there are two people in your family or twenty-four—blended, married, divorced, single, empty-nesters, co-parents, and everything in between—ALL families are important. Some kids are raised by a mom and dad, some are raised by two moms or two dads, while others are reared by grandparents, one mom, or one dad.

But let's face it: no family is perfect. And that's okay! All of us have arguments, drama, misunderstandings, and tough times—that's why it's important to remember we're all just doing our best. And deep down, we're all longing for the same thing: healthy, loving connections.

We strengthen these connections and create harmony in our homes with small, daily rituals like family dinners, hugs before bed, saying "I love you" as our kids leave for school, one-on-one chats and anything else we can squeeze in. Traditions like vacations, family parties, and date nights also strengthen our connections and build unity in our lives. And nothing can substitute for both quantity and quality time.

Using words and actions we can also teach our kids to love and appreciate *all* families in our communities. By teaching our kids to respect other families, whatever their make-up, we will teach our kids to value and prioritize our own families. It is crucial that our kids understand that families are the basic unit of society and therefore each of us must do our part to create a healthy home where kindness, respect, and hard work rule—a place where our family members can thrive.

- -

DISCUSSION QUESTIONS

👑 What is love? How do you know you are loved?

👑 What is marriage? Why do people get married? Why do they stay married?

👑 What does the word "family" mean to you?

👑 Who is your family?

👑 What makes some families different from others? How is your family unique?

👑 Is it ok for other families to have a different structure than ours? (for example: one parent vs. two; married vs. divorced; grandparents raising the kids vs. parents raising the kids)

- How do you show your family that you love them?

- Why do people get divorced?

- If Mom and Dad are divorced, does that mean we are not a family anymore?

- Do kids cause divorce? Is it ever their fault? (No! Divorce is a grown-up issue. Kids do not cause divorce.)

- What is a blended family? (After a divorce, people sometimes remarry and mix their families together!)

- What are some of the rituals, family sayings, and traditions in our family that make us unique?

- What are some new traditions or rules that might help our family get along better?

- What do you imagine your future family will be like? Do you want it to be like our family?

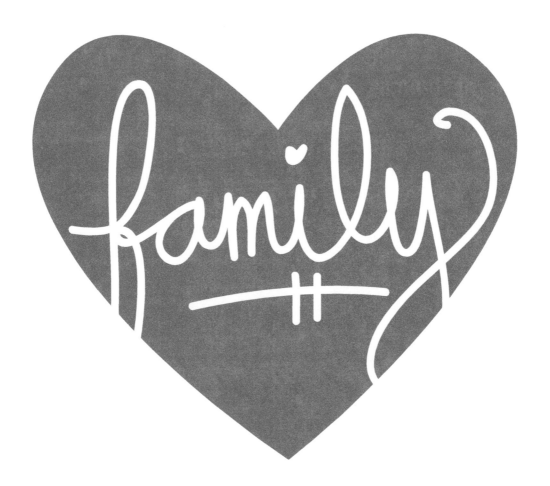

ACTIVITIES

Hold a Family Council

Plan a time that you and your family can meet together to discuss issues important to you. This family meeting may focus on serious topics like how to get along better, planning and saving for a family purchase, setting family goals, altering family rules, etc. Here are some guidelines to help you run a meaningful family council:

- Loosely plan what you would like to accomplish before the family meeting

- Turn off distractions and tune in to each other

- Start your meeting by sharing something positive

- Encourage discussion

- Make decisions together

- End with positive family time

Love Notes

Have each family member write a short note of love and gratitude to each member of the family. Provide paper, cards, and pens for each person. Give any other guidelines you think will help your kids to write heartfelt notes of kindness. Put a reminder in your phone to repeat this activity once every 4–6 months.

CITATIONS/RESOURCES

Alexander, D., et. al. (2016). *30 Days to a Stronger Child.* Rising Parent Media.

Educate and Empower Kids. (Sep. 8, 2018). For Parents: How to Have a Family Council. Retrieved from https://educateempowerkids.org/wp-content/uploads/2018/01/Family-Council-Lesson-Plan2.pdf.

Herring, H. and M. Bergman. (Dec. 5, 2018). Deeply Connecting with Our Kids: Moving Beyond "How Was Your Day?" Retrieved from https://educateempowerkids.org/6354-2/.

Loyd, K. (Aug. 31, 2018). Holding Family Meetings: A Necessity for Our Busy Families. Retrieved from https://educateempowerkids.org/5450-2/.

Park, C. (n.d.) 5 Things a Father Can Do to Increase His Daughter's Self-Worth. Retrieved from https://educateempowerkids.org/5-things-a-father-can-do-to-increase-his-daughters-self-worth.

Webb, J. (Sep. 7, 2018). Connecting Families through Daily Rituals. Retrieved from https://educateempowerkids.org/connecting-daily-rituals/.

17. HEALTHY SEXUALITY

Messages about sexuality are everywhere—plastered on billboards, blaring on the radio, and saturated in other mainstream media and the internet. Unfortunately, most of the information we are bombarded with on a daily basis is unhealthy and often inaccurate. In its most caustic forms, it may include **pornography**, rape, **human trafficking**, and other forms of sexual abuse.

As parents, it's our job to teach our kids the difference between these convoluted messages and healthy sexuality. In its honest, authentic form, **sex** is beautiful and healthy, and not something our kids should be ashamed of! As we teach our kids to love their bodies, they will be better equipped to reject false information they receive about sex through media and pornography.

The best thing we can do is create a safe place where we can have open conversations with our kids. As a result, they will be safer, more savvy, and better equipped against low self-esteem, sexual predators, and sexual abuse. That's a pretty tall order! But it all begins with simple, straightforward chats about healthy sexuality!

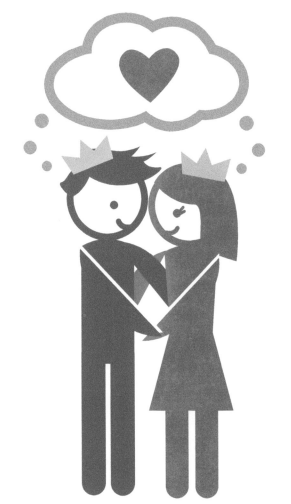

DISCUSSION QUESTIONS

- What is the difference between romantic love and the kind of love we might feel for a friend or family member?

- Why do we kiss and hug people we like and love?

- What are some different ways people show affection?

- Why does loving someone make people want to express those feelings in a physical way?

- What is **masturbation**?

- Is it ok for kids to masturbate?

- What is **sex**?

- What is **intimacy**?

- Have you heard anything about sex that you would like to talk about?

- Is it ok to talk about sex with your parents? Is it ok to talk about sex with your friends at school?

- If you have questions about sex, where should you go for answers? Is it a good idea to search for information about sex on the internet? Why or why not?

- When is the right time to have sex?

- Do you decide the next step in a relationship or does your partner?

- Why is it better to wait to have sex until you are in a committed relationship?

- Is it ok to have sex for purely physical satisfaction?

- Does sex feel the same for everyone?

- What is an **orgasm**?

- What is **consent**?

- Is it ok to stop having sex once you've started?

- What is rape? What is sexual abuse?

- If someone tries to touch your private parts, how can you tell them "no"?

- What should you do if someone touches your private parts? What if you know the person? If they ask you to keep it a secret, should you tell your parents anyway?

- What is the difference between good touch and bad touch?

- Do you have to let someone kiss or hug you just because they are your family?

- What is a sexual predator? Can other kids be predators?

DISCUSSING INSTINCTS THAT CAN KEEP YOU SAFE

Have you ever met a person that gives you a funny, uncomfortable feeling in your gut?

Predators will often use methods to groom children (and parents!) into a false sense of security, encouraging them to ignore those early warning signs. Teach your kids to recognize stress reactions, like butterflies in their tummy, jelly legs, goosebumps, sweaty palms, racing heart, nausea, or even diarrhea in extreme cases (Martin, 2016). These are reactions from our autonomic nervous system that warn us something is wrong, and they can help protect kids from abuse. Tell your kids to report to you if anything happens to them that causes these kind of reactions in their body.

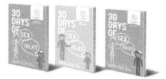

DISCUSSION FOR OLDER KIDS & TEENS

What are STDs and STIs? What are some ways to prevent them?

If you have been in a dating relationship for a long time, and your boyfriend or girlfriend wants to have sex, is it ok to say "no"? If you have different ideas on this topic, should you end the relationship or is it ok to stay together? Why or why not? Who decides the next step in your relationship? Is it okay to stop having sex once you've started?

CITATIONS/RESOURCES

Alexander, D. (n.d.). Talking with Our Kids about Masturbation—Without Shame! Retrieved from https://educateempowerkids.org/talking-with-our-kids-about-masturbation/.

Alexander, D. (n.d.). Talking with Our Daughters about Masturbation. Retrieved from https://educateempowerkids.org/talking-daughters-masturbation/.

Benuto, L. (n.d.). Healthy sexuality. Retrieved from https://www.mentalhelp.net/articles/healthy-sexuality/.

Educate and Empower Kids. (2015). *30 Days of Sex Talks: Empowering Your Child with Knowledge of Sexual Intimacy* (3 vols: For Ages 3–7, For Ages 8–11, and For Ages 12+). Rising Parent Media.

Fifty Shades is Abuse. (n.d.). National Center on Sexual Exploitation. Retrieved from https://endsexualexploitation.org/fiftyshadesgrey/.

Grover, L. (n.d.). How Teaching Healthy Sexuality Can Help Your Child Against the Predator, the Pressuring Partner, and the Prude. Retrieved from https://educateempowerkids.org/teaching-healthy-sexuality-can-help-child-predator-pressuring-partner-prude/.

Harkey, M. (n.d.). For Survivors of Sexual Abuse: How to Talk to Kids About Healthy Sexuality. Retrieved from https://educateempowerkids.org/survivors-sexual-abuse-talk-kids-healthy-sexuality/.

Hilton, C. (n.d.) Helping Children Develop Healthy Sexual Attitudes. Retrieved from https://educateempowerkids.org/4681-2/.

Martin, H. (2016). *Parents' Guide to Child Protection Education: How to Teach Body Safety and Abuse Prevention*. Safe4Kids.

Scott, A. (n.d.). Why We Need to Fight for Our Kids' Healthy Sexuality. Retrieved from https://educateempowerkids.org/why-we-need-to-fight-for-our-kids-healthy-sexuality/.

Van Orden, T. (n.d.) Talking with Your Teen about Sex. Retrieved from https://educateempowerkids.org/talking-teen-sex/.

18. LGBTQI ISSUES

LGBTQI: Lesbian, Gay, Bisexual, Transgender, Queer, Intersex (See Glossary for details)

We live in a world where ideas about sexual identity and gender identity are continually evolving—as evidenced by the ever-expanding acronym for LGBTQI issues. We are surrounded by ideas about sexuality in the news, mainstream media, and even on the playground. So we shouldn't be surprised when our kids bring home questions about LGBTQI issues at the dinner table.

We also need to accept and respect the fact that our children and their friends have different views or might make choices regarding gender and sexuality that we wouldn't make ourselves. How will we react if or when this happens? Will we knee-jerk with an attitude of fear or anger? Or will we create a safe place where we treat everyone with love and **compassion**? As parents, the choice is ours. And the time to prepare is now.

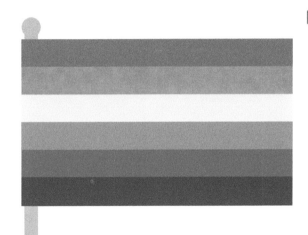

DISCUSSION QUESTIONS

🦋 What does LGBTQI stand for?

🦋 Do you know anyone who identifies as LGBTQI?

🦋 What does "gay" or "lesbian" mean? Is it appropriate to use these terms when discussing members of the LGBTQI community? What does "straight" mean?

🦋 How are gay people and straight people different?

🦋 How are those who identify as gay (or any of the other terms listed above) and straight people the same?

🦋 Do you believe it is right or wrong to identify as a member of the LGBTQI community?

🦋 Should these personal values affect the way we treat people who identify as LGBTQI?

🦋 Can LGBTQI people get married or have children?

🦋 If you wanted to come out as LGBTQI would you feel comfortable telling me? Who among your friends and family members could you tell?

🦋 Some people may use derogatory terms like "fag" or "dyke." Why is this destructive?

> How does **bullying** affect LGBTQI people? Have you seen any evidence of this at school or in the community?

> How can we show kindness and respect to everyone regardless of their sexual or gender identity?

ACTIVITIES

Role Play
Imagine that a family friend (a peer of one of your children) has told you that he or she has a same-gender attraction. What would you do? Role play at the dinner table. Start out with your child saying, "My friend [invent a fictitious name] has come out as [gay, transgender, etc.]." Go from there. Try to be real, and see where the conversation leads.

Current Events Discussion
Find a current event in the news about LGBTQI issues that you would like to share with your kids. Find a link to a news story or video clip about it, review it with your kids, and discuss the story with them.

CITATIONS/RESOURCES

Educate and Empower Kids. (2015). *30 Days of Sex Talks: Empowering Your Child with Knowledge of Sexual Intimacy* (3 vols: For Ages 3–7, For Ages 8–11, and For Ages 12+). Rising Parent Media.

Robinson, A. and M. Spears. (Jan. 9, 2019). Starting Conversations with Your Kids about LGBTQ Identities. Retrieved from https://educateempowerkids.org/starting-conversations-kids-lgbtq-identities/.

Robinson, A. and M. Spears. (Jan. 7, 2019). Guess Who's Coming to Dinner 2019. Retrieved from https://educateempowerkids.org/guess-whos-coming-dinner-2019/.

ADDITIONAL RESOURCES

Center For Disease Control and Prevention. LGBTQ Youth Resources. Information from the CDC, other government agencies, and community organizations that outlines the health needs of LGBTQI youth, which can differ from those of their peers. https://www.cdc.gov/lgbthealth/youth-resources.htm

Child Welfare Information Gateway. Resources for Family of LGBTQ Youth. Resources to help families support their lesbian, gay, bisexual, transgender, and questioning (LGBTQ) youth; understand what to expect; and learn how to talk about a number of issues that may be impacting them. https://www.childwelfare.gov/topics/systemwide/diverse-populations/lgbtq/lgbt-families/

LEAD with Love: Additional Resources for Parents and Youth. Information and resources for parents of gay, lesbian, bisexual, and transgender children. http://www.leadwithlovefilm.com/parents/files/resources.pdf

John Hopkins Medicine. Tips for Parents of LGBTQ Youth. An article outlining information regarding communication, education, bullying, and other topics, as well as other resources for parents of lesbian, gay, bisexual, transgender and questioning children. https://www.hopkinsmedicine.org/health/articles-and-answers/ask-the-expert/tips-for-parents-lgbtq-youth

Supportive Families, Healthy Children. A booklet from San Francisco State University designed to create open communication and provide resources and help for families with lesbian, gay, bisexual and transgender children. http://familyproject.sfsu.edu/sites/default/files/FAP_English%20Booklet_pst.pdf

SELF IMPROVEMENT

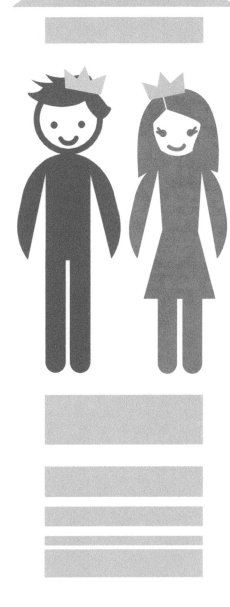

Each of us is born with a potential for greatness. Throughout our lives we develop our intellect, talents, and individual gifts. But it's not just success that creates greatness. It is our failures, our missteps, and our trials that teach us, humble us, and cause us enormous growth.

We can encourage our kids to try new things, step out of their comfort zones, and prepare for the difficult times that will inevitably come their way. They need to know that they CAN do hard things! This doesn't have to happen serendipitously. We can teach our kids how to talk about tough topics, face challenges, and plan and prepare for success.

19. OVERCOMING FEARS

Everyone gets scared sometimes—adults too! It is a natural part of life that allows us to be tested and develop courage. We must be willing to take risks and be willing to fail. We must learn through experience that risk and failure alike teach their own lessons.

It can be tempting however to avoid the things we fear. But avoidance prevents us and our kids from learning that scary situations or places are not dangerous.

To overcome our fears, we often have to *take the initiative*—this means not waiting for others to solve our problem. Taking initiative in our lives doesn't necessarily mean undertaking huge tasks. Instead, taking initiative might look like doing our homework without being asked, remembering to do our chores, offering to help a sibling, or even just raising a hand in class to answer a question.

Talking about our fears is a great start. Tell your kids about some of the fears you had as a child, as a teen, and that you have now. Discuss ways you faced your fears and overcame them. Did it happen with small steps and practice? Did overcoming the fear involve looking at things in a new way? Did you ask for help in order to get through your fear? Don't forget to share what people, experiences, or other things helped you find courage.

- -

DISCUSSION QUESTIONS

- How do we develop fears?

- Some people have real issues with anxiety that require medical attention and/or medication. How is this different from normal fears that people can overcome with hard work or support from loved ones?

- What are some things people fear? (public speaking, being different, feeling embarrassed in front of others, being alone, starting something new, moving to a new place)

- What do you fear? What is a fear you have faced? How did you overcome your fear?

- What are some obstacles that keep us from trying new things?

- Is there anything in your life that you want to try but feel nervous to start? What's holding you back?

- What are some small steps you can take to help you overcome your fears?

- How do we distinguish between real fears and the ones we create?

- Are you afraid of what others will think or say?

- What advice would you give to a friend who is scared to try something new?

- How can you maintain your self-confidence in the face of people or situations that make you question your worth?

- What do people mean when they say you can't be brave without feeling fear first?

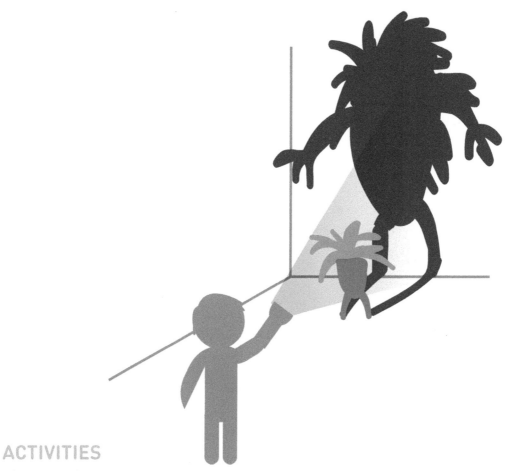

ACTIVITIES

Share a Talent
Challenge your child to pick a talent they have and display it or share it with others. It can be telling jokes, doing magic tricks, drawing a picture, or doing a headstand. Keep it simple. Have them document how they felt as they shared this ability with others.

Recognizing and Letting Go of Fear
Have your child choose an adventure and write his or her worries or fears about that adventure on a piece of paper, then throw it away or burn it. Teach your child to let go of their worries or fears as the paper disappears. If possible, take your child to experience the adventure they identified.

20. FINDING REAL JOY

Everyone has had fun sometime in their life—whether it's laughing at a great joke, feeling the thrill of a roller coaster, shopping for a treat, or hanging out with friends.

But **joy** is more precious and requires a little more effort. People feel joy in different ways. Some describe joy as a feeling of contentment, peace or gratitude, or a sense that one's life is good, meaningful, and worthwhile.

Even though it usually requires work and comes over time, joy is more lasting and is felt on a deeper level than happiness. Part of this is due to the fact that understanding joy often involves also understanding things like sadness and pain. As we live through hard things and experience a full range of emotions, we learn to appreciate the opposites in life. A person cannot understand good health if they have never been sick, nor can they really know what light is if they have never been in the dark. The same can be said for sadness and joy.

We can also experience joy when we DO healthy things. Being creative, working, exercising, giving of your time and abilities, and trying to make a difference in the world all bring joy. People who are great listeners, who share their possessions, serve with their time and energy, and take time to learn and empathize with others are generally more joyful people.

Make a goal to take the initiative in helping others and being grateful for what you have and who you are. Find opportunities to create joy in your life by being with the people you love and enjoying simple things. Take time to be still and feel joyful.

DISCUSSION QUESTIONS

- What do you like to do for fun? What are some things that bring you **joy**? How can you tell the difference between joy and fun?

- Do you find joy in being with others or having quiet solitude?

- Do you find joyful experiences when you are creating something? Working with your hands? Learning something? Doing something physical like playing a sport? Doing something adventurous?

- Can you describe one of the most joyful moments or times in your life? (Perhaps it's not a one-time event.)

- Why do we need sadness in order to understand real joy? If we never experienced sadness, could we really have joy?

- Have you heard the expression, "Find joy in the journey"? What does this mean?

- Have you heard, "It's better to give than to receive"? How is this a statement about joy?

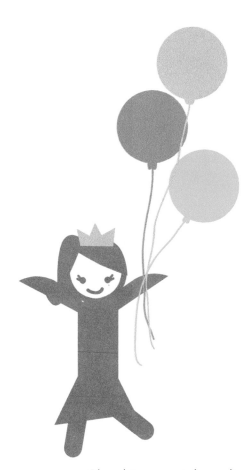

ACTIVITIES

Inside Out

Watch the movie *Inside Out*. Discuss the need for both joy and sadness in our lives. Ask your kids the following questions:

- Could Riley really feel joy if she had never experienced sadness in her life?

- What went wrong when the character Joy tried to force happiness into every experience for Riley?

- Although we try to avoid sad or disappointing experiences in life, why are they necessary?

Social Media Fast

We are so heavily influenced by what we "should like/do/have/buy" that this so often is not in line with what truly brings us joy. For many of us, social media has become a necessity in our day. If ditching social media altogether is not an option, think about how you can cut down on it. For example:

- Checking social media sites just twice a day: once mid-morning, so you're not starting your day with social media, and again late afternoon.

- Opting for a maximum of two portals of instant messaging communication that friends and colleagues can contact you on. Some employers and friends contact us through text, email, WhatsApp, Skype, direct Instagram messaging, and regular phone calls. This can be far too overwhelming!

- Choose the people you "follow" or who appear in your feed wisely. If you like to get your daily fix of what's happening around the globe—whether it be in world affairs, fashion or self-development—opt for those who inspire you, not those who bring you down.

CITATIONS/RESOURCES

Alexander, D., et. al. (2016). *30 Days to a Stronger Child*. Rising Parent Media.

Fearnley, R. (Sep. 1, 2015). Joy vs. Happiness. Retrieved from https://www.psychologies.co.uk/joy-vs-happiness.

21. KEEPING OUR "ACCOUNTS" FULL

Every person has various internal qualities that need to be balanced in order to function. When we work to develop these qualities, we not only function–we thrive! We learn, we adapt, we grow, we share, and we find our greatness.

Each of these qualities or "accounts"–the social, the emotional, the spiritual, the physical, and the intellectual–is important and necessary to live a healthy, balanced, and strong life.

We can think about developing these qualities in terms of maintaining an "account balance." Our goal is to keep our accounts full and balanced in order to be healthy. Typically, when one account is empty we borrow from other accounts. For example, when a person feels lonely or upset, he may overeat to try to fill his account–borrowing from his physical account to fill his emotional account. When several accounts are low, we usually experience anxiety, sadness, and even depression or physical illness.

DISCUSSION QUESTIONS

- How does keeping our accounts full help us to be truly healthy?

- We have a physical, social, emotional, intellectual, and spiritual account. What are some things we can do to fill our physical account? (eating healthy, exercising, avoiding harmful substances, etc.)

- What are some things we can do to fill our social account? (being a great friend, treating others with respect, creating healthy boundaries, etc.)

- What are some things we can do to fill our emotional account? (having empathy, giving or receiving a hug, using **positive self-talk**, etc.)

- What are some things we can do to fill our intellectual account? (taking time to be creative, learning, experimenting, being curious, etc.)

- What are some things we can do to fill our spiritual account? (having a belief system, being grateful, sharing in a community, serving others, etc.)

- What are some behaviors or situations that can deplete our accounts? (stress, procrastination, being around negative people, being bullied, excessive screen time, overwork, not getting the rest we need, etc.)

- What can we do about people who seem to drain or deplete our accounts?

- How do we think and feel when our accounts are full? How do we think and feel when our accounts are empty?

- Does the status of our accounts affect our actions?

ACTIVITIES

Science Experiment

Show your kids two soda cans. One should be closed and full of soda. The other one should be empty. Discuss the importance of keeping our "accounts" full and how having full accounts helps us to withstand pressure and stress. Have your child try to crush the full soda can with one hand. (They will find this nearly impossible.) Then have your child crush the empty soda can. Discuss situations, people, and other things that can deplete our accounts and what we can do to keep our accounts well balanced.

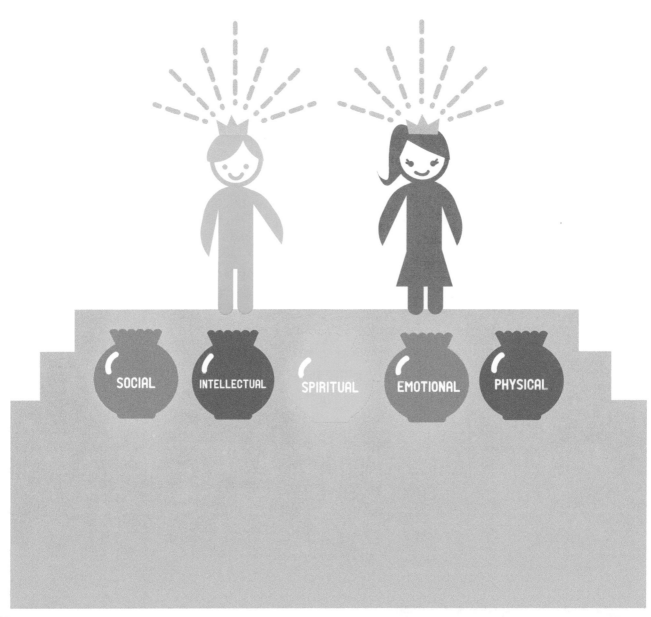

Depositing Compliments

Gather your family or a group of your child's friends together. Give everyone a piece of paper and a pencil.

1. Tell each person to write their name at the top of the page.

2. Have everyone pass their paper to the person on their right.

3. When they receive a new paper, they should write something they admire or like about the person at the top of the page.

4. Continue passing the papers to the right and writing compliments on each person's paper until the papers have traveled around the entire circle.

5. Once everyone has their own paper back, have each person read the list of compliments aloud.

At the end of the exercise, point out that everyone feels better about themselves and gets a small "deposit" to their accounts when they receive compliments. Challenge everyone to stop negative self-talk by remembering this list!

CITATIONS/RESOURCES

Alexander, D., et. al. (2016). *30 Days to a Stronger Child.* Rising Parent Media.

King, K. (n.d.). Tick Tock Goes the Clock: Finding Balance Between Social Media and Family Time. Retrieved from https://educateempowerkids.org/5103-2/.

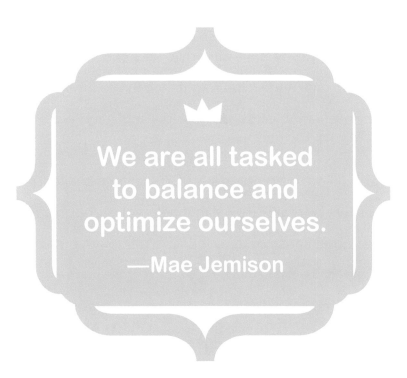

We are all tasked to balance and optimize ourselves.

—Mae Jemison

22. ADVERSITY AND HARD TIMES

Everybody will experience **adversity** at some time (or many times) in their life. We may lose a loved one, have trouble in school, get diagnosed with a physical or mental illness, experience divorce, or have another tough problem. But even in the most challenging times, we have the opportunity to make choices. We can choose how we will react, how we will treat others, what we will say, and what attitude we will bring to each situation.

Over the years, I have heard three survivors of the Holocaust speak about their experiences. Each of them said that they knew no matter how hard their life was, no matter how terrible the conditions, no matter how powerless they felt, no one could take their thoughts from them. And no one could take their faith.

Knowing this, they realized in their darkest hours that they could keep going, even if it was minute to minute or just getting through the next hour. This was their gift: this way of thinking and behaving is what created and sustained their strong, survivor spirit.

Let your kids know there is no "right" way to approach difficult life experiences. Most of the time we are right in the middle of a challenge before we realize what is happening. But there are some skills that can help get us through. **Optimism**, **positive self-talk**, having a sense of humor, and a belief system have all been proven to help people through hard times (Alexander, 2016).

- -

DISCUSSION QUESTIONS

🔱 What is **adversity**?

🔱 What is a challenge you have already overcome in your life?

🔱 What are some challenges you might face in the future?

🔱 From your observations, how do your parents handle adversity?

🔱 What does it mean to be optimistic? Do you face challenges with **optimism**?

🔱 What is **positive self-talk**? How can it help you through a rough day?

🔱 How does a good sense of humor help a person in good times and bad?

🔱 Sometimes, particularly during hard times, we might say, "I will be happy when___ is done," or "If only I could_____, then I would be happy." What is the problem with this type of thinking? How can we choose to be positive or feel content even when times are tough?

♛ Why does a belief in God or a "higher power" help some people when they are dealing with very difficult circumstances?

ACTIVITY

Sharing Life Experiences
Share with your kids one of the most difficult experiences in your life. Tell your kids how you got through it. What did you do right? What would have made it easier? What do you regret?

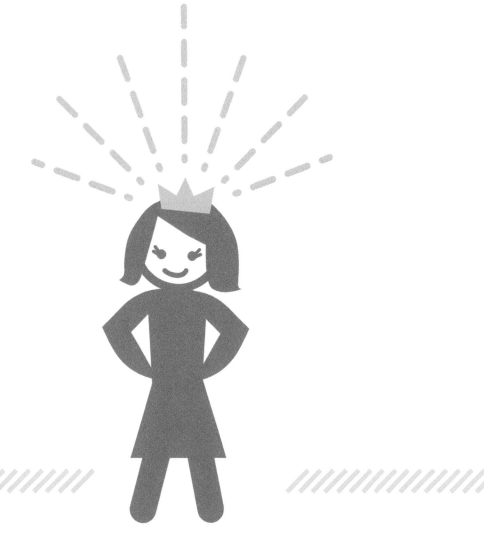

CITATIONS/RESOURCES

Alexander, D., et. al. (2016). *30 Days to a Stronger Child.* Rising Parent Media.

23. ADDICTION AND CONNECTION

Sometimes a person may ingest a substance that induces pleasure (like drugs or alcohol), and then develop a need for that substance. This is called **addiction**. But addiction doesn't just refer to substances. Neurological research shows how addiction to food, gambling, video gaming, and **pornography** can affect the brain–literally changing the way it works. This need can become a compulsion that interferes with ordinary life responsibilities such as work, relationships, or health.

Addictive tendencies exist in everyone. People can even become addicted to generally positive behaviors like exercise, work, sex, shopping, and bargain hunting. New research shows that *feeling connected* is the best way to heal from addiction. Healthy connections and happy relationships can also help us steer clear of addiction in the first place (Hari, 2015). As Johann Hari said, "The opposite of addiction is not sobriety. The opposite of addiction is connection."

DISCUSSION QUESTIONS

- What are some substances that people can become addicted to?

- What are some behaviors that people can become addicted to?

- What is the difference between prescription drugs and recreational drugs?

- All of us have addictive tendencies. What can we do to identify those addictions that each of us is most susceptible to?

- What would you do if you felt like you were developing an addiction? Where would you go for help?

- Has anyone at school ever offered you a substance you weren't sure about? If this ever happened, what would you do?

- Who are the most important people in your life right now? Who helps you to feel loved? (These are the people you are connected to.)

- What are some ways we can be more connected to one another?

- People often overeat, do drugs, excessively game, watch porn, and do other unhealthy things when they are bored, lonely, sad, depressed, or stressed out. What do you do when you feel these emotions? What can you do to avoid these unhealthy habits?

- Can you remember the last time you felt really angry or really sad? What did you do? How did you cope? Have you ever heard the term **coping mechanism**?

ACTIVITIES

Healthy De-stressing
When your child returns from a stressful situation like school, try employing a de-stressing technique before your child heads for the fridge, TV, or digital device. Offer to play a board game or go for a walk. Use healthy, enjoyable ways to de-stress and your child will be less likely to turn to mindless, unhealthy, addictive activities to wind down and relax.

Change Together Challenge
Most of us have one or more negative habits that need replacing, so join your child in a challenge to change! The point is to connect with your child as you challenge yourselves to change together. Remember, when he or she feels connected, they are empowered to avoid turning to unhealthy sources to feel that connection.

DISCUSSION FOR OLDER KIDS & TEENS

Addiction causes people to lose control of their behavior and do things they would not usually do. Sometimes this can lead to poor life choices that affect not only the person who is addicted, but also their loved ones and society as a whole. With guidance from a parent or trusted adult, choose one or more of the following topics, and do some research about them: drunk driving, drug abuse, celebrities who have died from drug overdose, addiction recovery programs, U.S. Opioid Epidemic. (See Resources below.)

Vaping is a habit that is becoming very popular among teens and young adults—even in middle school. Do you think this is an addictive behavior? Would you vape if it was offered?

CITATIONS/RESOURCES

Alexander, D., et. al. (2016). *30 Days to a Stronger Child*. Rising Parent Media.

Benson, M. (n.d.) How Parents Can Help Children Overcome Porn Addiction. Retrieved from https://educateempowerkids.org/parents-can-help-children-overcome-porn-addiction/.

Educate and Empower Kids. (May 5, 2018). Lesson: Talking to Your Kids About Addiction. Retrieved from https://educateempowerkids.org/wp-content/uploads/2017/06/Addiction-Lesson-Plan2-2.pdf.

Educate and Empower Kids. (Jan. 8, 2017). Addictive Behavior and the Brain's Reward Circuit. Retrieved from https://educateempowerkids.org/addiction-and-the-reward-circuit/.

Hari, J. (2015). Everything You Think You Know about Addiction is Wrong [Video File]. Retrieved from https://www.ted.com/talks/johann_hari_everything_you_think_you_know_about_addiction_is_wrong?language=en.

Hilton, D. H. and C. Watts. (2011). Pornography Addiction: A Neuroscience Perspective. *Surgical Neurology International*. Vol. 2, no. 19. Retrieved from https://www.ncbi.nlm.nih.gov/pmc/articles/PMC3050060/. doi: 10.4103/2152-7806.76977.

National Institute on Drug Abuse. Teens and E-cigarettes. Retrieved from https://www.drugabuse.gov/related-topics/trends-statistics/infographics/teens-e-cigarettes.

U.S. Department of Health and Human Services. (2019). What is the U.S. Opioid Epidemic? Retrieved from https://www.hhs.gov/opioids/about-the-epidemic/index.html.

24. SETTING GOALS

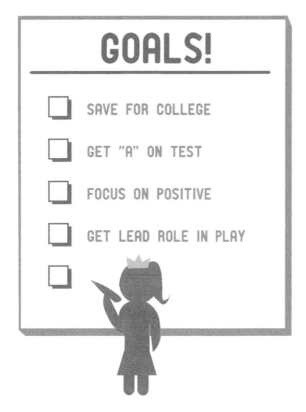

When you teach your kids how to set and achieve **goals**, you are giving them a skill that not only brings success, it brings emotional well-being. A person can have physical, emotional, intellectual, social, financial, and even spiritual goals. Creating goals can be fun and gives us new purpose.

Goals should be specific and have a meaningful purpose that you think will improve you or your family in some way.

As you set out to make a goal that motivates, make it with the positive in mind. Remember to make it "SMART": Specific, Measurable, Attainable, Relevant, and Time Bound. Definitely write it down. And always make a plan!

Teach your kids to follow through and stick to their goals, especially when things get tough. You will both enjoy great satisfaction as your children set goals, achieves them, and build character in the process.

DISCUSSION QUESTIONS

- Have you ever set a goal before?

- What goals do you have for yourself in school?

- What kind of career do you want when you grow up?

- What kind of person do you want to be when you grow up? What kind of lifestyle would you like to have? (home, family, world-traveler, etc.) What goals might help you achieve that lifestyle?

- What other long-term goals do you have?

- -

- What are some SMART goals (Specific, Measurable, Achievable, Rewarding, and Time Bound) that we can make as a family?

- What are some challenges we might face as we try to achieve our goals?

- If we experience difficulties while pursuing a goal, what can we do to get back on track?

- Who are some people that can help us with our goals?

- What are some small goals we can start with?

- How can we make goals fun?

- What obstacles might we face as we try to accomplish these goals?

- What benefits could we experience if we are successful in keeping these goals?

ACTIVITIES

Individual Goals
Challenge your child to set a goal and work on it for a month. Outline some small daily or weekly steps to help your child achieve their goal. For example, if you have a child that is starting at a new school, you might suggest that he set a goal to make one new friend each week or each month. Daily and weekly steps might involve introducing himself or saying hello to someone new once a day.

Family Goals
As a family, have each member set a goal to replace something that isn't working very well in your lives with a better choice. Write the goal down and set small daily and weekly goals to change your habit. Give yourselves time to accomplish the goal and recognize your small achievements along the way.

CITATIONS/RESOURCES

Alexander, D., et. al. (2016). *30 Days to a Stronger Child*. Rising Parent Media.

Parents Magazine. (n.d.). How to Teach Kids Perseverance and Goal-Setting. Retrieved from https://www.parents.com/parenting/better-parenting/style/how-to-teach-kids-perseverance-goal-setting/.

Park, C. (n.d.). Goals: Starting the Year Right. Retrieved from https://educateempowerkids.org/goals-start-year-right/.

25. MONEY MANAGEMENT

Every child will use money at some point in their childhood and they will generally learn how to actively spend and save money from the example set by their parents. As parents, we should take a look at our spending, saving, and investment practices to see what habits we are passing on to our kids through our words *and* our example.

Discuss what an allowance is and why you give your child one or why you don't. Explain what saving is and why delayed gratification and saving is critical to their future well-being. Take a few minutes to talk about some of the healthy and unhealthy choices you have made over the years with money and emphasize some of the strategies you used as you adjusted to adult financial concerns like college tuition, bills, sharing an account with a spouse, etc.

Share your experience with debt, worrying about money, and overspending. Talk about both giving and receiving.

DISCUSSION QUESTIONS

- What have you learned from your parents about money? Is money something to worry about? Is it something to argue about? Is it something that only concerns adults? Is it a tool? A curse? An asset?

- Benjamin Franklin said, "Money never made a man happy yet, nor will it. The more a man has, the more he wants. Instead of filling a vacuum, it makes one." What does this mean?

- Why is earning money more rewarding than just having someone give it to you?

- Why is earning our own money and paying for things ourselves good practice for adulthood?

- What are some helpful or meaningful ways we can spend money?

- What can you buy with $20? With $1,000? With $100,000?

- What are some fun ways we can spend money?

- When does fun spending become wasteful or unhealthy?

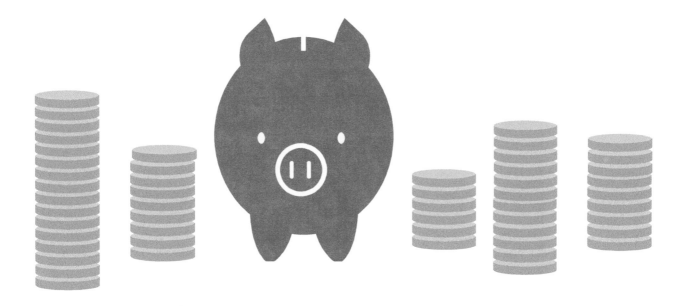

Some people go shopping when they are bored, lonely, stressed out, or depressed. Why might this turn into an unhealthy habit?

How much money should we save? What are the benefits of saving?

Why can saving money be a challenge?

What is credit and what are credit cards used for?

What is **interest**? How does interest work? What is compound interest? What are ways you can make interest work for you? What are ways interest can work against you?

If you wanted to buy a house that cost $400,000.00, how much money would you need to have saved in order to get a loan from a bank?

Many people are paying off loans for their education or a house. Is it okay to go into debt for these kinds of things? What are some kinds of loans or debt we should *avoid*?

What does it mean to "live *within* your means"?

What are the consequences of "living *above* your means"? Why do so many people do it?

What is the difference between a *want* and a *need*?

- What does it mean to **invest** money? What are some things a person can invest in? (stocks, mutual funds, property, businesses, etc.)

- Have you heard the saying "The love of money is the root of all evil"? What does this mean? Is it true?

ACTIVITIES

Open a Savings Account
Take your child to your local bank and open a savings account with them. Explain what **interest** is. If possible provide motivation for your child to continually earn and add money to their account (like a matching program—for every dollar they put in their account, you will add 25 cents to their account until they reach $500—or something similar).

Stock Market Game
As a family, choose to follow five to ten stocks for a set number of weeks. Use Monopoly money or something similar to "buy" stocks. Discuss the benefits of long-term and short-term investments. Look at each of your stocks each day (or every week) and determine which ones to keep and which ones to "sell." At the end of the game, talk about your successes, your failures, and what you learned together.

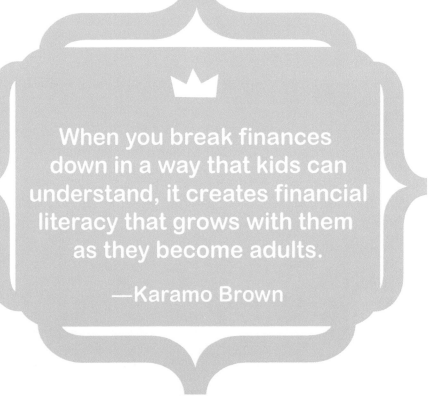

When you break finances down in a way that kids can understand, it creates financial literacy that grows with them as they become adults.

—Karamo Brown

DEEPER TOPICS

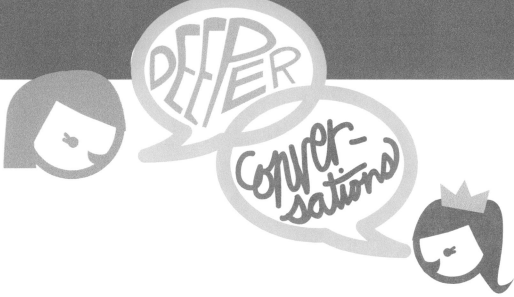

Because we live in a fast-paced, image-obsessed culture, it's easy to get overly busy, caught up in shallow pursuits, or mindlessly move from task to task, activity to activity, or scroll through social media without examining what we are doing or why.

Each of us needs to take a step back and ponder on the deeper experiences of life to really study out the principles and people that make our lives meaningful and give us hope. We can ask questions like:

- Why are we here?
- Why should I choose to be generous or kind?
- What can I do with the knowledge and power I have?
- How can I help others who suffer?
- How can I overcome difficult times?
- What happens when we die?

We must learn to slow down, develop a sense of **integrity**, and consider what really matters to us and whether we are living a life consistent with our values. As you work through the following topics, you can determine what topics you need to cover more thoroughly and what topics of your own to add to help your kids become functioning, compassionate adults who thrive, even in tough times.

26. AGENCY

Agency is often described as the ability to make choices. But it's so much more than that. It is the freedom of knowing that you are responsible for yourself, your choices, and your actions. Even when you're in a class that is difficult, working with people that are rude or unhelpful, or experiencing terrible circumstances (like a death or divorce in your family), you can choose your thoughts, your attitude, and your actions.

As you get older, you are given more choices, but you will also better understand the short-term and long-term effects of those choices. Our choices shift from topics like what toys to play with or what to eat and soon become choices about which friends to have, how much effort to put into school, and what you want to be when you grow up. Most importantly, you will realize that you can actually choose to be content or happy even during hard times. You can choose to work hard when others are not. You can choose to stand up to a bully even if you feel scared.

We make many choices every day. We always have choices! But we cannot always choose our consequences.

When you are an *agent*, you realize your power and potential. You can be an agent of change, choosing to help others and bring change to your family, your school, and/or your community.

Sometimes we confuse freedom with agency. But they are different concepts. **Freedom** refers to having rights and not being in slavery or bondage. Agency is the ability to know truth and to act on that knowledge. Agency can also refer to exerting power or choosing your thoughts and actions.

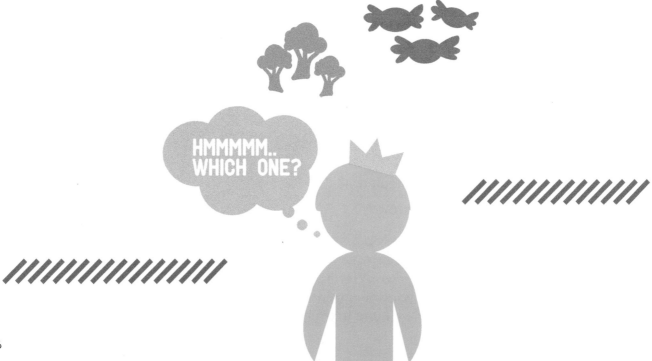

HMMMMM.. WHICH ONE?

👑 What is **agency**? How do you get agency?

👑 Our freedoms can be taken away (ex: going to prison). But, is it possible for our agency to be taken away?

👑 A lot of small choices can have a big impact. What are some of the small choices we make each day? How does the way we choose to talk to ourselves impact our feelings and other choices?

👑 How does the way we choose to treat others affect both us and them?

👑 What are some of the important choices you make each day?

👑 We can use our agency to help and lift others. What are some of the powerful things we can do to serve or support others?

- -

ACTIVITY

We Need Knowledge to Have Agency
Write various tasks on slips of paper large enough to be easily read. Place these in a bowl and have your kids choose a slip of paper while blindfolded. Then let them choose with their eyes open, looking at what's written on the slips of paper. Ask them which way is more likely to result in a choice they want.

Discuss that while they may get what they want without looking, the chances of satisfaction are much greater when they can see the choices and know what they are choosing. In order to make wise choices, we must have knowledge about our options and their related consequences. Our ability to choose well improves as we learn which consequences come with which choices.

- - - - - - - - - - - - - - - - - - - -

Sarah's Choice
Read the following story and then discuss the following questions:

Sarah played volleyball throughout her childhood. Her parents both played and sometimes coached her team. As a teenager she thought about playing other sports and wondered if she only played volleyball because her parents played and pushed her to be on a team. Should she try out for the team again this year? Or do something different? She talked with her parents and friends about her concerns. After a lot of thinking, she decided that she really loved playing volleyball. It was a great workout, and she loved playing with her teammates and scoring points. Since deciding for herself that she enjoyed the game, playing volleyball has been even more fun and rewarding for Sarah.

Why is it *freeing* to know that you make a choice because you want to and not because someone told you to? Why is it better to take responsibility for or to "own" our choices?

Why does it feel so good to know "I am _____ because I choose to be"?

Choosing Peace
When we understand our agency, we discover great power in our own choices. How can we choose to be at peace in the following circumstances? What actions can we choose?

- Being sick with a cough and runny nose

- Not being able to play outside because of rain or snow

- Having your phone taken away

- Getting a low grade on a test

- Losing something important

- Having a good friend move away

- A parent losing their job

DISCUSSION FOR OLDER KIDS & TEENS

Read a summary or all of the book, *Man's Search for Meaning* by Viktor Frankl. Discuss agency and the power of our thoughts. Ask your kids where they find meaning in their lives.

CITATIONS/RESOURCES

Teaching Children to Use Agency Wisely. (n.d.). Retrieved from https://www.lds.org/ensign/1988/10/teaching-children-to-use-agency-wisely?lang=

We Can Choose. (n.d.). Retrieved from https://www.lds.org/manual/family-home-evening-resource-book/family-home-evening-lessons/lesson-eight-we-can-choose?lang=eng.

27. INTEGRITY

Integrity: To be honest and have strong moral principles. The quality of being truthful, dependable, and constant.

Integrity is usually accompanied by choices. For instance, we might choose to play with a particular friend, help a neighbor, or take the garbage out without being asked.

We sometimes think that integrity is natural and easy, but being honest and having integrity take practice. We need to practice having integrity in easy *and* difficult situations. Small lapses in integrity lead to bigger lapses. For example, if we are willing to copy someone's homework, then we are more likely to cheat on a small quiz or on a big test.

Sometimes it can be tempting to say or do things online we wouldn't normally do. Even when people are rude to us online, we must remember that there is a real person on the other side of the computer screen and treat others just how we would in person.

Even though it is very important to choose wisely, all of us will make foolish choices. But we can pick ourselves up and choose to do better. When we do this, it is vital that we acknowledge our mistakes to ourselves AND to those we have wronged or been dishonest with. We can make the decision to change. We can stop a bad habit that threatens our integrity. We can make a commitment to tell the truth in all circumstances, to be authentic online, and to be kind to everyone—not just our friends and people we admire.

We can choose to have integrity even if we might get into trouble, look bad in front of others, lose money, get a low grade, or worse.

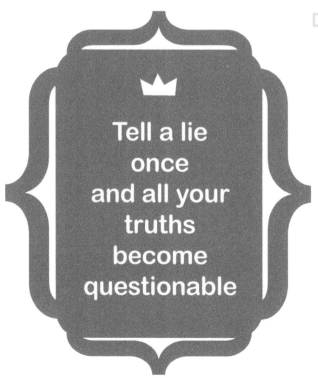

Tell a lie
once
and all your
truths
become
questionable

DISCUSSION QUESTIONS

👑 What does it mean to have **integrity**?

👑 Integrity is a pattern of thought and behavior, but what does it look like?

👑 We make lots of choices each day (what to eat, what to say, how to react to kind or rude people, how to deal with a dilemma). What do our choices tell others about us? What do our choices say about who we really are?

👑 Integrity comes when we consciously choose who we want to be. By choosing our actions carefully—both in real life and online—we develop into the people we want to become. Do our everyday choices affect us and others?

- Sometimes we **rationalize** our decision to outright lie or tell only a part of the truth by telling ourselves that "no one will know" or "everyone does it." What other things might we say or think to **justify** not having integrity?

- How is being rude or unkind on social media showing a lack of integrity?

- How can we show integrity at school? Online? At work?

- - - - - - - - - - - - - - - - - - - -

- Are there ever circumstances where it is okay to lie?

- Who are the people in your life that have integrity and who you trust?

- What does it mean to be honest with yourself?

- Why would you want your family, friends, and teachers to think of you as a person of integrity?

- Some people say that you have a responsibility to yourself to develop your talents and abilities. If you are showing integrity to yourself, how hard would you work in school? With your talents?

ACTIVITIES

Family Code of Ethics
Develop a **code of ethics** together as a family. What does your family believe? How do you want your family system to be run? How will your actions reflect integrity both in real life and online? Define your own thoughts and feelings and compromise with each other until you all have a system of beliefs that represents all members of the family.

Decide Ahead of Time
Discuss situations where a choice needs to be made. For example: cheating on an exam, finding lost money, speeding on the highway, underage drinking, speaking up for others, reaching out to a new person, responding respectfully to others. Discuss the benefits of deciding NOW how to respond in these situations.

- - - - - - - - - - -

CITATIONS/RESOURCES

Alexander, D., et. al. (2016). *30 Days to a Stronger Child.* Rising Parent Media.

28. SPIRITUALITY IN RELIGION

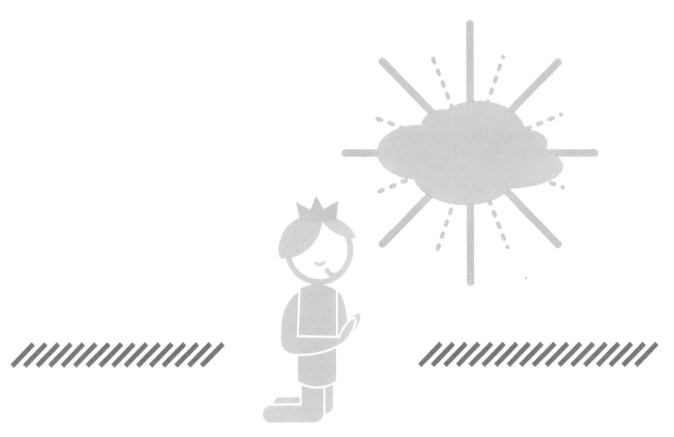

Developing a sense of **spirituality** does not necessarily mean subscribing to a particular religious view, but instead is a process to help you develop tools that can be used when you face challenges, pain, and other difficult emotions in your life. Having a sense of your spirituality can help you to have the strength to deal with such challenges in a positive and healthy way, rather than a destructive way.

There are many ways a person can cultivate their spirituality. One way is for people to find meaning in their lives and connect to the world in a positive way. It can also involve "slowing down, sitting still, and taking the time to listen" (Alexander, 2016). Showing gratitude, choosing to make positive changes in one's life, showing love towards others, spending time in nature, and joining in a religious congregation are all great ways a person can develop their spiritual side.

Being involved in a **religious** community is a very common way for people to nurture their spirituality. These communities work together to accomplish goals that are larger than each individual. Many people enjoy building friendships there, doing service for others, learning various self-improvement techniques, and learning more about religious texts like the Torah, the Koran, the Bible, or various sutras, Vedas, or hymns.

DISCUSSION QUESTIONS

👑 What does it mean to believe something? What are some things that you believe? Can you think of some ways your beliefs shape your world?

👑 Do you only believe in things you can see? How could someone believe in something they can't see?

👑 How can your beliefs make you stronger?

👑 Does spirituality mean that we have to believe in a god or religion? What's the difference between spirituality and religion?

👑 Did we exist before we were born? Why are we on the earth? What happens when we die?

👑 Do you think there is a God? If so, where does God live? How can God be "everywhere"? Why does God allow **suffering**?

👑 Why do we to go to church? Why do our friends go to a different church?

👑 Who wrote the Koran? The Torah? The Bible? Who invented religion?

///

ACTIVITIES

Learn about Different Religions
Through online, reputable resources or by talking to friends and neighbors who practice a particular faith, find out what it means to be Jewish, Hindu, Buddhist, Muslim, Christian, Jain, Sikh, Bahá'í, Taoist, etc. You may wish to find out about specific sects of these religions (Orthodox Jew, Sunni Islam, Shia Islam, one of the four major sects of Hinduism, etc.). Christianity is popular in U.S. Culture. Find out about people who belong to various Christian denominations such as the Catholic Church, Episcopal, Baptist, Church of Jesus Christ of Latter-Day Saints, etc.

Practicing Gratitude
Gratitude is a specific spiritual practice basic to every belief system. Set a goal as a family to practice active gratitude each day. Active gratitude signifies consciously setting aside a few moments for reflection and expressions of gratitude during specific times throughout the day. For example, you may wish to practice active gratitude before a meal, before bed, after waking up, or at another time throughout the day. You might choose to share with each other verbally or you could even write down your ideas on a whiteboard or journal. Talk to each other and encourage each other to remember!

CITATIONS/RESOURCES

Alexander, D., et. al. (2016). *30 Days to a Stronger Child*. Rising Parent Media.

29. SUFFERING

It is highly likely that you will never meet anyone with an "easy" life (or at least anyone who thinks they have an easy life). Everyone has problems and challenges. All of us will face things that scare us, many of us will struggle with an **addiction** or long-term illness, and all of us will lose somebody close to us.

Not all **suffering** is bad. Each of us will face challenges and struggles—this is where we grow, change, and become better, stronger people. Often, as we suffer, we build **resilience**. However, there are some people—many of them children—who face truly harsh life experiences. They may live in poverty, be surrounded by disease, war, or death, and be the victims of truly evil acts.

Much of suffering is caused by people making selfish choices. Wars are almost always started by such selfish choices. Greed and the struggle for power are huge factors in what motivates individuals, families, tribes, and whole nations to exploit or harm others. These actions then lead to the destruction of cities, villages, and peoples' lives. Death and disease closely follow in these circumstances.

People who are suffering deserve our **empathy**! This is not to say that we always try to take away other people's problems, resolve their issues for them, or enable someone who is addicted to a substance! But we can often be helpful in a variety of ways, and we can always try to imagine what their experience is like and try to "walk with them."

- -

DISCUSSION QUESTIONS

👑 What causes **suffering**? (death, disease, war, politics, **apathy**, evil, etc.)

👑 What might be an example of someone's own actions causing their own suffering?

👑 If someone causes their own suffering, does that mean we don't need to help them?

👑 Some suffering is caused by nature or accidents and is generally unavoidable. Can you think of an example of this? (a hurricane destroying someone's home, a healthy person getting cancer, falling down the stairs and getting a life-altering injury, etc.)

👑 What is **apathy**? How does our apathy lead to other people's suffering?

👑 We sometimes ignore the suffering of people who live far away. Why is that?

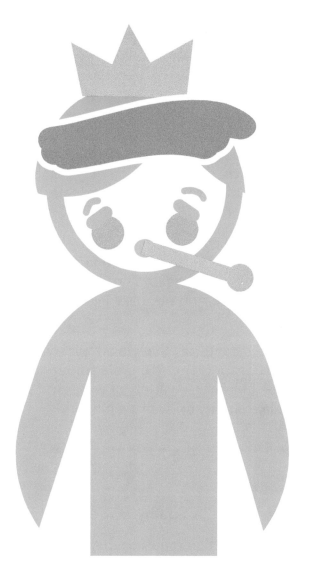

- We sometimes dismiss others' suffering because we think we can't do anything about it. We can't stop all suffering in the world, but what are some things we can do to prevent people from suffering?

- We often cannot take away someone's pain, but we can "walk with them" and be supportive. What does this mean?

- How can we help people without enabling a problem that they themselves perpetuate?

- If there is a God, why does He allow so much suffering to happen in our world?

- Where does evil come from?

- What is **empathy**? How can we develop more empathy within our family? Within our school or community? With people living in another part of the world?

- Do we know anyone who is suffering right now? How can we be helpful to them?

- What can you do if you are suffering? Who can you turn to?

ACTIVITIES

Use the News

Watch the news or visit a news website every evening for three days. Discover what is happening around the country and around the world. Discuss what is going on and if there are people suffering. Is there anything you can do to help? Can you donate to the Red Cross? Can you write a letter or email to people working in national or foreign governments? Can you share what you have learned with friends or on social media to bring awareness to the problem? Determine what you can do, then do something!

Develop Empathy
Have your child choose a friend or family member that they would like to feel more empathy towards. Encourage regular interactions with this person. After each interaction, discuss your child's feelings for this person and help your child identify respective needs after spending time with this person. Help your child identify ways in which she could offer assistance or otherwise show them that she cares for them. Make this a regular endeavor.

Discuss Suffering
Discuss the fact that *not all suffering is bad.* Each of us will face challenges and struggles—this is when we grow, change, and become better, stronger people. Encourage each family member to share a difficult experience in their life that has made them stronger or changed their life for the better.

CITATIONS/RESOURCES

Alexander, D., et. al. (2016). *30 Days to a Stronger Child.* Rising Parent Media.

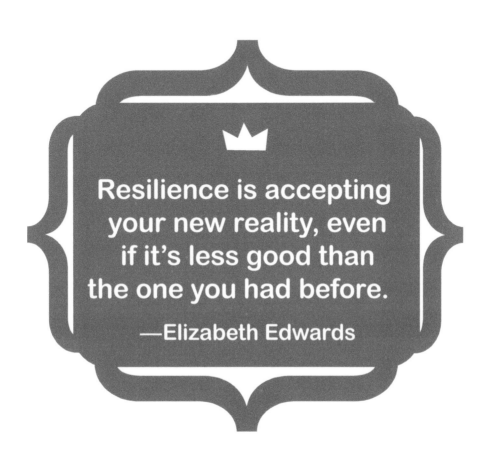

Resilience is accepting your new reality, even if it's less good than the one you had before.

—Elizabeth Edwards

30. DEATH

Death: The end of life.

Death can be a fascinating or sometimes terrifying topic for children. There are so many unknown factors for them and for adults. Especially for this generation, death seems more mysterious than it did for our great-grandparents or even our grandparents, who experienced the death of family members and loved ones much more frequently. Since most of us experience a relatively low mortality rate in our cultures, death is often not discussed or explained as readily.

Helping kids understand death will help them understand *life* better. It will give them the words to talk about loss, sadness, mourning, and other topics that can be difficult for kids–and adults–to articulate. Having open discussions about death can also help our children prepare for the inevitable losses they will experience in their lives.

- -

DISCUSSION QUESTIONS

👑 Does everyone die? Do we know when we will die?

👑 Will we be together when we die?

👑 What does "dead" mean?

👑 Why do pets/animals/living things die?

- -

QUESTIONS YOUR KIDS MIGHT HAVE

👑 Will they be back?

👑 Was it my fault?

👑 Did they die because they did something bad?

👑 Did it hurt? Does death hurt?

👑 Why do people die?

👑 Is death forever?

👑 When do people die?

👑 What happens after death? Where do you go?

👑 Do people have a soul? What is a soul?

👑 If they go to heaven, then why are they buried?

👑 Can they see me from heaven?

///////////////////////////////////////

ACTIVITIES

Remembering a Loss
Gather a few photos of a friend or family member who has passed away. Talk about what this person was like and what you loved most about them. Explain what it was like for you when you lost this person. Discuss some of your mourning process and how you found peace. Openly share your beliefs regarding what you think happens when someone dies.

Write Your Epitaph
In discussing death, it's important to acknowledge that one's body—whether it is buried or cremated—is just one part of an individual. Ask each member of your family what they want to be remembered for, then have everyone decorate a tombstone on a piece of paper and write their epitaph based on their response. Or, simply have everyone write down what they want said about themselves when they die, then share and respond.

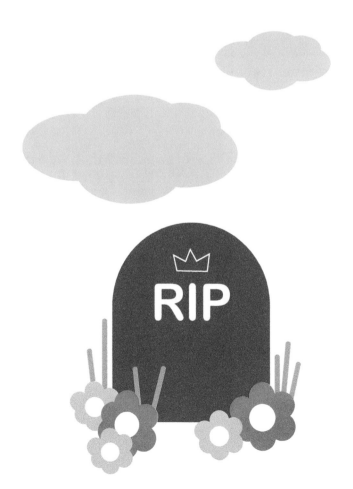

GLOSSARY

Addiction: A condition that results when a person ingests a substance (for example, alcohol, cocaine, nicotine) or engages in an activity (for example, gambling, gaming, pornography use, shopping) that can be pleasurable but the continued use/act of which becomes compulsive and interferes with ordinary life responsibilities such as work, relationships, or health.

Adversity: Unfavorable times; a condition marked by misfortune, difficulties, stress, or sadness.

Agency: The ability to know truth and to act on that knowledge. Agency can also refer to exerting power or choosing your thoughts and actions.

Algorithm: A step-by-step method of solving a problem. It is commonly used for data processing, calculation and other related computer and mathematical operations. An algorithm is also used to manipulate data in various ways, such as inserting a new data item, searching for a particular item or sorting an item.

Apathy: Showing a lack of concern, often by ignoring or neglecting.

Artificial Intelligence (AI): A branch of computer science, sometimes called machine learning, where computers and other devices understand their environment, learn from experience, and take actions that maximize their chances of successfully achieving their goals.

Bullying: Unwanted, aggressive behavior among school aged children that involves a real or perceived power imbalance. The behavior is repeated, or has the potential to be repeated, over time. Bullying can be done through threats, physical or sexual violence, harassment, persistent efforts to embarrass or humiliate, relentless teasing, etc. It can occur in person or behind the screen of a phone, computer, or another device.

Capitalism: An economic and political system where a country's trade, industry, and financial growth are controlled by private owners for profit, rather than by the state.

Carbon Footprint: The total amount of greenhouse gases produced to directly and indirectly support human activities, usually expressed in equivalent tons of carbon dioxide (CO_2). Your carbon footprint is the sum of all emissions of CO_2 (carbon dioxide) which were induced by your activities in a given time frame.

Code of Ethics: A set of rules, principles, values, and commitments that a person, family, or organization agrees to and follows.

Compassion: A feeling of deep sympathy and sorrow for another who is stricken by misfortune, accompanied by a strong desire to alleviate the suffering.

Consent: Clear agreement or permission to permit something or to do something. Consent must be given freely, without force or intimidation, and while the person is fully conscious and cognizant of their present situation.

Coping Mechanism: Using certain behaviors or distractions to deal with, get through, or avoid stressful, embarrassing, sad, or unpleasant experiences. These can be positive (reframing a situation, talking it out, exercising) or negative (using illegal drugs, taking one's anger out on someone else, self-harm).

Cyberbullying: Bullying that takes place online through social media, gaming sites, platforms, text, or instant messaging. Electronic devices typically used are cell phones, tablets, or computers.

Death: The end of life. Being dead.

Deconstruct (Media): To break down an ad, movie, commercial, song, or other media into pieces to see what the real message is.

Deliberate: Consciously doing something, being mindful. Thinking before you act.

Digital Citizenship: Developing skills and knowledge to use the Internet and other digital technology competently, particularly to participate responsibly in social and community activities.

Empathy: The feeling that you understand and share another person's experiences and emotions; the ability to share someone else's feelings.

Environmental Issues: Problems with the Earth's systems (air, water, soil, etc.) that have developed as a result of human interference, lack of proper planning, or exploitation of the planet.

Feminism: The belief that women should be allowed the same rights, power, and opportunities as men. It is also a political and social movement that seeks to solidify this belief.

Freedom: The state of being unrestricted and free, free from slavery. Being able to claim rights and privileges.

Global Warming: A gradual increase in the overall temperature of the earth's atmosphere generally attributed to the greenhouse effect caused by increased levels of carbon dioxide, chlorofluorocarbons, and other pollutants.

Globalization: The spread of economic, political, and social ideas and interactions across cultures and all over the world.

Goal: Something you are trying to achieve; an aim or desired result.

Human Trafficking: Human trafficking is modern-day slavery and involves the use of force, fraud, or coercion to obtain some type of labor or commercial sex act.

Integrity: To be honest and have strong moral principles. The quality of being truthful, dependable, and constant.

Implicit Bias: Any unconsciously held set of associations about a social group. They are the product of learned associations and social conditioning. They often begin at a young age, and most people are unaware that they hold them.

Intimacy: Generally a feeling or form of significant closeness. There are four types of intimacy: 1) physical intimacy (sensual proximity or touching), 2) emotional intimacy (close connection resulting from the honest exchange of thoughts and ideas), 3) cognitive or intellectual intimacy (resulting from the honest exchange of thoughts and ideas), and 4) experimental intimacy (a connection that occurs while acting together). Emotional and physical intimacy are often associated with sexual relationships, while intellectual and experiential intimacy are not.

Intentional: Doing something with purpose, being deliberate.

Interest (Money): Money paid regularly at a particular rate for the use of money lent, or for delaying the repayment of a debt.

Invest (Money): Putting time or money into something, hoping that there will be returns greater than what was originally put in.

Joy: A deep, lasting feeling of peace, well-being, and happiness. Joy is developed over time and usually involves us giving a part of ourselves to gain it.

Justify: To try to prove or show that you are right or reasonable.

LGBTQI Terms

> **Lesbian**: A word used to describe women who are sexually attracted to other women.

> **Gay**: A term used to describe people who are sexually attracted to members of the same sex. The term "lesbian" is generally preferred when talking about women who are attracted to other women. Originally, the word "gay" meant "carefree"; its connection to sexual orientation developed during the latter half of the 20th century.

Bisexual: Sexual orientation in which one is attracted to both males and females.

Transgender: A condition or state in which one's physical sex does not match one's sense of one's gender identity.

Queer: A historically derogatory term against people who were homosexual, an identity in which Gay and Lesbian individuals have taken back so they could take the negativity away from the word and use it to say they were proud. It is also an umbrella term for sexual and gender minorities who are not hetero-sexual.

Intersex: A general term used for a variety of conditions in which a person is born with reproductive or sexual anatomy that doesn't seem to fit the typical definitions of female or male. For example, a person might be born appearing to be female on the outside, but having mostly male-typical anatomy on the inside.

Masturbation: The self-stimulation of the genitals in order to produce sexual arousal, pleasure, and orgasm.

Optimism: A feeling or belief that good things will happen in the future.

Orgasm: The rhythmic muscular contractions in the pelvic region that result from sexual stimulation. Characterized by a sudden release of built-up sexual tension (climax) and by the resulting sexual pleasure.

Pornography: The portrayal of explicit sexual content for the purpose or intent of causing sexual arousal. In it, sex and bodies are commodified for the purpose of making a financial profit.

> *Easy definition for young kids*: Pictures or videos of naked or partially clothed people. There is usually sexual activity in it.

Positive Digital Citizenship: Using technology to enhance your family, school, and community through tolerance, kindness, authenticity, and ingenuity.

Positive Self-Talk: Talking to oneself—either out loud or silently—in a positive, kind manner.

Prejudice: Disliking a group of people or things without good reason; a preference for one group over another.

Racism: The idea that one's own race is superior and has the right to dominate others or that a particular racial group is inferior to the others.

Rationalize: An attempt to explain or justify a behaviour or an attitude with one or more reasons, even if these are not appropriate.

Religion: A set of beliefs concerning the cause, nature, and purpose of the universe. Religion usually involves devotional and ritual observances, and often contains a moral code governing the conduct of human affairs.

Sex (Sexual Intercourse): Sexual activity, also known as coitus or copulation, which is most commonly understood to refer to the insertion of the penis into the vagina (vaginal sex). It should be noted that there are a wide range of various sexual activities and the boundaries of what constitutes sexual intercourse are still under debate.

Social Class: A division of a society based on social and economic status. Four common social classes informally recognized in many societies are: (1) Upper class, (2) Middle class, (3) Working class, and (4) Lower class.

Spirituality: The quality of being concerned with the human spirit or soul as opposed to material or physical things.

Stereotype: A widely held but oversimplified image or idea of a particular type of person or thing. It is a preconceived notion, especially about a group of people. Many stereotypes are racist, sexist, or homophobic.

Suffering: Experiencing pain, distress, or extreme hardship.

Terrorism: Violence—or equally important, the threat of violence—used and directed in pursuit of, or in service of, a political aim.

Tolerance (Addiction): A state in which one no longer responds to a drug or stimulus. A higher dose is required to achieve the same effect.

Tolerance (Kindness): Sympathy for or patience with beliefs and practices that differ from or conflict with one's own.

GLOSSARY CITATIONS

Berghoef, K. (n.d.). What Does Implicit Bias Really Mean? Retrieved from https://www.thoughtco.com/understanding-implicit-bias-4165634.

All About … (n.d.) Definition of Religion. Retrieved from https://www.allaboutreligion.org/definition-of-religion-faq.htm.

Interest, s.v. Oxford Dictionaries. Retrieved from https://en.oxforddictionaries.com/definition/interest.

Kenton, W. (Dec. 13, 2018). Capitalism. Retrieved from https://www.investopedia.com/terms/c/capitalism.asp.

MacMillan, A. (Dec. 7, 2018). Global Warming 101. Retrieved from https://www.nrdc.org/stories/global-warming-101.

National Institute on Drug Abuse. (n.d.). 6: Definition of Tolerance. Retrieved from https://www.drugabuse.gov/publications/teaching-packets/neurobiology-drug-addiction/section-iii-action-heroin-morphine/6-definition-tolerance.

Time for Change. (n.d.). What is a Carbon Footprint—Definition. Retrieved from https://timeforchange.org/what-is-a-carbon-footprint-definition.

Religion, s.v. Dictionary.com. Retrieved from https://www.dictionary.com/browse/religion.

Russell, S. and P. Norvig. (2003). *ARTIFICIAL INTELLIGENCE: A Modern Approach*. Prentice Hall.

Ward and Antonia. (Jun. 4, 2018). How Do You Define Terrorism? Retrieved from https://www.rand.org/blog/2018/06/how-do-you-define-terrorism.html.

Techopedia. (n.d.). What is an Algorithm? Retrieved from https://www.techopedia.com/definition/3739/algorithm.

What Is Bullying? (n.d.). Retrieved from https://www.stopbullying.gov/what-is-bullying/index.html.

What Is Human Trafficking? (Oct. 17, 2018). Retrieved from https://www.dhs.gov/blue-campaign/what-human-trafficking.

What is intersex? (n.d.). Retrieved from http://www.isna.org/faq/what_is_intersex.

THANK YOU FOR READING!
IF YOU ENJOYED THIS BOOK, PLEASE LEAVE A POSITIVE REVIEW ON AMAZON.COM.

FOR GREAT RESOURCES AND INFORMATION, FOLLOW US ON OUR SOCIAL MEDIA OUTLETS:

Facebook: www.facebook.com/educateempowerkids/

Twitter: @EduEmpowerKids

Pinterest: pinterest.com/educateempower/

Instagram: Eduempowerkids

SUBSCRIBE TO OUR WEBSITE FOR EXCLUSIVE OFFERS AND INFORMATION AT:

www.educateempowerkids.org

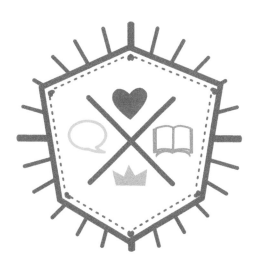

Printed in the USA
CPSIA information can be obtained
at www.ICGtesting.com
LVHW071256300524
781813LV00017B/348